MUSIC
MEDICINE

Christine Stevens, MSW, MT-BC

MUSIC
MEDICINE

The Science and Spirit of
Healing Yourself with Sound

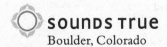

SOUNDS TRUE
Boulder, Colorado

Sounds True, Inc.
Boulder, CO 80306

Published 2012

Cover design by Jennifer Miles
Book design by Jennifer Miles and Dean Olson

Stevens, Christine, 1964–
Music medicine : the science and spirit of healing yourself with sound / Christine Stevens.
    p. cm.
Includes bibliographical references.
ISBN 978-1-60407-799-5
1. Music therapy. 2. Music — Psychological aspects. I. Title.
ML3920.S815 2012
615.8'5154 — dc23

                                2011052524

eBook ISBN: 978-1-60407-831-2

10 9 8 7 6 5 4 3 2 1

Dedicated to Connor Sauer,
beloved mentor, teacher, and spirit-mom

Immerse yourself in the rapture of music.
You know what you love. Go there.
Tend to each note, each chord,
Rising up from silence and dissolving again.

Vibrating strings draw us
Into the spacious resonance of the heart.

The body becomes light as the sky
And you, one with the Great Musician,
Who is even now singing us
Into existence.

—SUTRA 18, *VIJNANA BHAIRAVA TANTRA (THE RADIANCE SUTRAS)*,
TRANSLATION BY LORIN ROCHE, PHD

CONTENTS

Foreword

A song can awaken the soul. When we listen to music, we might get goose bumps, breathe more deeply, or feel a flood of emotions that brings us to tears. Old memories might surface. The human response to music is indicative of how deeply music touches the mind, body, heart, and soul. Most of us love music, but have we really considered using its depth as a tool for stress reduction, health, and wellness? Even more, have we considered its great potential to transform communities and the planet?

I first met Christine Stevens while teaching at a retreat near Nashville, Tennessee. Within minutes, she had more than ninety people drumming, singing, harmonizing, and then sitting in silence together. The diverse audience that day included people in recovery from drug and alcohol addictions, therapists, and community members. Christine guided the group through experiences of the four elements of music—rhythm, melody, harmony, and silence—and created a parallel between those elements and the four directions of the medicine wheel. Through her workshop, we learned how to consciously listen to music and to freely make music.

The retreat participants came alive, smiles were contagious, and the rhythms united us all. There was a shared sense of freedom and joy, and a renewed connection to the inner pulse of life within. I sensed the credibility and creativity of Christine's method of musical engagement and her specific applications of music for body, mind, heart, and soul. The transformation was evident that day as we crossed a threshold from music lovers to creators of our own music. Now through *Music Medicine,* you can make this transformation, too.

Music is one of the oldest forms of spiritual medicine known to humanity. If you look at ancient texts from most traditions, they have musical notations next to them. The Torah, for example, is not only read—it's also chanted. In ancient Greece, Pythagoras of Samos taught his students how certain musical chords and melodies could produce a wide range of responses within the body. The shamanic healers of tribal cultures use drumbeats and chanting to support healing experiences. It's no different in our society, where groups of people gather to chant melodies and drum rhythms to open doorways into other realms. In the experience of music, thoughts can take a backseat, and the essence of peace can be attained.

As a scientist, I have long observed a phenomenon—sound and melody, used as a form of meditation, turn off the thinking mind. I always suspected there must be research showing which brain mechanisms are at play in this process. And in fact a surprising amount of music research is emerging from leading laboratories and universities, much of it using brain-scan equipment and cutting-edge genetic analysis.

This book examines these scientific findings in depth and brings forth a profound conclusion: that the gift of music isn't necessarily about what music *does* for us; it's about what music *un-does* in us. When we engage music on a deep level, whole parts of the brain are turned off in an activation and deactivation pattern. Christine finds that this neurological system is replicated at the genomic level; musical participation switches off genes that signal stress alerts to our minds and bodies.

Medical and scientific literature is finally catching up to the ancient wisdom of music medicine and further supporting how music is an evidence-based technique for mind, body, heart, and soul health and healing. Strikingly, many studies show that music is an inherent part of who we are as human beings, woven into our very genomic code and evident even in newborn babies. This explains why music tugs at our heartstrings and strikes a chord in our souls.

Years ago, when I ran a stress disorders clinic at one of the Harvard Medical School teaching hospitals, I often told my clients that they were already whole and healed. The purpose of the tools we gave them in our clinic was to peel away the layers of stress that covered their naturally wise, peaceful, and compassionate hearts. Most of us carry some form of musical wound: a sense that we are untalented, perhaps from a childhood music teacher telling us we should lip-sync in the choir concert. Christine helps us peel off those layers and discover our inner "musical spirit." She allows us to awaken the music within for healing, connecting, harmonizing, and center-ing—skills much needed in the world today. In *Music Medicine,* she provides tools and techniques to bring music and sound into our lives through an abundance of guided practices.

In this way, Christine's approach is also practical. There has been a dramatic rise in the use of music to treat stress conditions in everyone from returning veterans and trauma survivors to overworked employees to people suffering from depression. I have extensively researched the all-too-common phenom-enon of "burnout" and have found that high levels of stress are a major factor. Likewise, I have found that resilience in the body, mind, and spirit naturally and sometimes dramatically occurs when individuals include stress-reducing activities in their lives. It is more important than ever to find affordable, simple, enjoyable strategies to reduce stress, strengthen our immune system, and build a sense of community with others. Music—when approached through the lens of empowerment, simplicity, creativity, and calm—can provide the sup-port we need in life's challenging moments and can become part of our daily routine for spirituality and health.

Christine's passion for her work and her curiosity about the healing and spiritual power of music have brought her to many unique places, from the sweat lodges of the Lakota to the war zones of Iraq. Her experience is the foundation from which she teaches. Her insights, stories, and scientific updates give us the sense of the ancient wisdom of music's power to heal, and her abil-ity to communicate her knowledge gives us a direct way to apply this wisdom to modern-day life. Enjoy this powerful path for your own musical healing— through the joy, and the great peace, of music.

Joan Borysenko, PhD
Author of *Minding the Body, Mending the Mind*

Acknowledgments

I thank the muse that illuminated this understanding and inspired this project.

Thanks to the team that worked to create this book: my agent, David Nelson, and editor, Florence Wetzel; Jeff Newman, my personal editor, who held space as we corralled ideas; and my content editor, Christoffer de Graal of Moving Sound in the United Kingdom, whose artistic heart brought depth and the distillation of key concepts in the dance of words that is this book. I also thank research assistant Becky Human, editor Jean O'Sullivan, graphics guru Drai Turner, and my assistant Agate Dawson. Thanks to all the Sounds True artists who allowed their recordings to be part of the playlists for each chapter. Thanks to the first cohort in the inaugural four-week Music Medicine course, which helped me shape the book's material as they grew into an ensemble of rhythm, song, harmony, and silence. And to the Sonic Beauty Circle, which has gathered at my home for a decade of ceremony and healing.

I am grateful for the Iraq drum-circle team: Z. Melinda Witter, Lydia Shaswar, Noaman, Mohammed, Kurdistan Save the Children, Jihad, Raz, Briyar, The Illuminators, Constantine Alatzas, Mark Montgyierd, and Craig Woodson. It was Mark's original medicine wheel diagram of our drum protocol that began to illuminate the connections that created this book. Thanks to our sponsors—National Association of Music Merchants (NAMM), Remo Drum Company, Rex Foundation, Mickey Hart, Kieron Sweeney, Musical Missions of Peace, and the Ocean of Gratitude Cruise.

Thanks to my council of cultural music experts, including Mark MaKai's Lakota music, Richard Rudis's Tibetan sound healing, Kim Atkinson's Afro-Brazilian ceremonial drumming, Gayan Gregory Long's Sufi and Buddhist understanding, Anton Mizurak's wisdom of India and Tibet, Stephanie Buffington's tribal music tours, Cameron Powers and Kristina Sophia's *tarab* of the Arab world, Michael Bourdet's DJ song support, and Kimber Godsey's mystery voice. I felt your support and wisdom pulsing through me with each beat of the keypad.

I thank Kathy Hull, who spent a whole year guiding me through the medicine wheel based upon Angeles Arrien's book *The Four-Fold Way*. And the uncanny coincidence that it was her brother, Arthur Hull, who taught me drum circles and the great mantra, "1–2—make up your own!" Woven together, their synergistic teachings brought the spirit and sound to life in music's medicine wheel.

I thank the spiritual guidance of Connor Sauer, founder of Long Dance; Uncle Manny Eagle Elk Council Pipe Sandoval and Uncle Peter Catches *Zintkala Oyate* of the Lakota Nation; Michael Bernard Beckwith, founder of Agape International Spiritual Center; Lorin Roche, meditation coach and translator of *The Radiance Sutras*; Berenice Andrews, teacher of the shamanic path; and Don Campbell, author and path-setter of sound and music heal-ing. I am grateful for key resources on the spirituality of music written by Hazrat Inayat Khan, Sri Chinmoy, and Paramahansa Yogananda. I thank my soul sister, Tina Landrum, for our rhythms of friendship and poetry, and Dan Cartamil, for our joyous musical sharing and soul-filled harmonies.

I'm grateful for the mentoring and dedication to excellent scientific contributions of Barry Bittman, MD, of the Yamaha Music and Wellness Institute. Dr. Bittman has been an inspiration of collaboration, focus, and dedication in his pioneering research in mind-body medicine and music. I thank Michael Thaut, PhD, at Colorado State University for the scientific foundation to build models of evidence-based music therapy.

I thank my family: My sister, Joy, whose dance, rhythm, and song bring joy to my heart. My dad, brother Owen, and all my muse-filled nieces and nephews—Ellie, Philip, Keira, Max, and Caden, who get to play music together in our three-generation family drum circles.

Lastly, I thank all the locations that hosted me while I wrote this book: May's Hollow in Encinitas, Paula Jean's dome in Joshua Tree, The Old Bear Bed and Breakfast at Mount Pinos in Los Padres National Forest, Coyote Canteen in Frazier Park, Stevenson Ranch, and the Remo Recreational Music Center in North Hollywood.

Prelude

This book is an invitation to take part in making your own music and to share it more widely in the healing that is taking place on the planet. Even though music is already in you, this book is a guide to remembering, reconnecting, and discovering the healing benefits of sound.

This is the story of an ancient artifact—or perhaps a fact of art—that has underscored thousands of years of humanity's development: the medicine of music. This treasure has been with us since the beginning of time. No war can destroy it. No one religion can claim it. Mystics of different faiths have heard its song, shamans have traveled its rhythmic beats to invisible realms, and healers have carried its tune to wounded souls. It is present in the symphony of the notes of our lives, the harmony between people, and the inner music that is unique to each person as a living instrument of his or her own song.

In the poorest lands, indigenous people who have "nothing" are shining with musical spirit, dancing and singing together. They know the secret. Most of the world has figured out this prescription for happiness, a pathway to healing that is embodied in music's medicine.

I want to serve as your guide to discover music's medicine—the sound, play, passion, and pause are waiting for you, a sonic remedy composed at the core of your being. I will take you through the four elements of music's medicine—rhythm, melody, harmony, and silence—with guided practices that show you practical ways to orchestrate healing and wholeness in your life and in the lives of those you serve. Then we'll move inward to the fifth element, which is the music within you, a quintessence that blends all four elements into the human instrument. Finally, we'll explore how music's medicine can orchestrate change in the world and for the planet.

This is a book that sings. Free online music playlists offer a soundtrack to the teachings on the groove, song, harmony, and silence within you. If you are in the fields of education, therapy, health care, or personal coaching, the guided practices can augment your work. If you are a parent looking to give your children the creativity and expression of music, you can incorporate the practices into your family life. If you are a musician, you can become more well rounded and create music that resonates more deeply from your soul.

This book is about a paradigm change. It's not about being taught music; it's about music teaching us. It's not about practicing music; it's about music as practice. It's not about talent; it's about truth. It's not only about loving music; it's about living music. It's about finding your way into a "sound" health strategy that is joyful, creative, harmonious, and fun.

My Quest for Harmony

I spent years in higher education, getting my master's degrees in both music therapy and social work, where I was taught theory, research, and practice. But my greatest education came through traveling. My work in training drum-circle facilitators and leading drum circles in places of war and tragedy took me to many places: Asia, Europe, Latin America, South Africa, Russia, and Iraq, to name a few. Making music with people of diverse cultures that preserved the traditions of sound and music for healing burst my heart open. I found such a rich heritage of music; even in places of great poverty and war, the songs, rhythms, and dances continued. My experiences opened my soul to the power of music cultures that are still preserved on the planet today.

When I paused and reflected on the lessons of my life, I looked at the common threads among these rich, yet very different experiences. I wanted to understand what the heartbeat of a powwow drum at a Lakota ceremony had in common with women chanting to celebrate the anniversary of the end of apartheid in South Africa; what singing to Hurricane Katrina survivors in New Orleans had in common with leading drum circles for peace building in Iraq. What were the common themes that transcended location, people, and culture and created sacred and healing musical experiences? The answers pointed toward the four elements of music, which independently hold unique healing properties.

Let me share with you some highlights from my life that were guideposts in the composition of this model of music's medicine.

In 2005, I traveled as a speaker on the Japanese Peace Boat to South Africa and Namibia. We were part of the ceremonies acknowledging the ten-year anniversary of the end of apartheid. While there, I led a drum circle and even met Archbishop Desmond Tutu. We went by boat to the Port of Walvis Bay, Namibia, where I took my drum to a poor village of tin-roofed homes. Hearing my drumbeat, an elder pulled out two spoons and started to play. No words were exchanged, only the energy of our drum-and-spoon-slapping groove. Even without drums, the rhythms of Africa were bursting in expression. The magnetic energy of rhythm drew others, and before I knew it, children were forming a circle around us.

One child with a deformed leg limped over and, to my amazement, started to sway and dance to the beat. He became a different boy; his body moved more fluidly and joyfully, a complete change from the difficult dragging stride he had used to join us. He moved to the center of our circle and continued to dance to the rhythms and the encouragement of the people. Without instruments, the bodies were the drums, dancing to the rhythm. I was discovering how rhythm is the medicine for the body.

Years before, while performing with Up with People in the former Soviet Union during the Mikhail Gorbachev era, I found myself joining an unforgettable demonstration of freedom by the Russian people, who were just beginning to experience free speech. I stood in a Moscow square, joining hundreds of people in singing "We Shall Overcome." A great sense of oneness permeated the crowd as this anthem of the American civil rights movement gave voice to the Soviet people's deep desire for freedom.

The heart's longing for freedom may be best expressed in song. The Russian people's call for revolution was amplified and synergized in the music. I saw that a song unites people, speaks the heart's language, and performs a kind of alchemy that transforms oppression to hope. I realized how melody is the medicine for the heart.

Everything I'd learned and taught in my life culminated in 2007, when I was invited to lead the first drum-circle training in an Iraqi war zone.

In a five-day workshop, my colleagues and I trained Iraqis from different language and religious groups on how to lead drum circles for conflict resolution and peacemaking. We met in a building that had once been a torture center during Saddam Hussein's regime, but which was now converted into a youth activity center.

The Kurdish and Arab trainees began to play their traditional instruments, sing songs, and even dance over the groove of the drum circles. I realized I was in a music culture in which there was no separation between drum, song, and dance. The result was a sacred space where opposing groups began to share cultural songs, rhythms, and dances with their former enemies. In the birthplace of civilization, music literally created harmony between conflicting groups and brought hope, peace, and healing to the wounds of genocide and the history of war. I was discovering how harmony is the medicine for the soul.

My global experiences in peace building were reflected back in my own spiritual quest. Even though I had spent years playing music for different religious groups—from playing organ for a Pentecostal church to drumming at the Agape International Spiritual Center—there was a deeper yearning in my spirit to come into direct contact with the Divine. My efforts at meditation grew frustrating because I have a very busy mind. But I persisted and learned to listen to the silence between the breaths, between the beats, and between the notes. Through chanting and mantra practices, I began to cultivate a silence that guided me to peace. Silence was the medicine of music that taught me to quiet my mind.

My most mystical experience of music's medicine happened in an unexpected moment while I was resting in a Japanese hotel, exhausted by the humidity and heat of a hot August day. As I lay on the bed, something strange happened; I began to hear my breath as if it were music. There was a rhythm in my inhale and in my exhale and a perfect balance in the pauses between my breaths. My heart felt filled with song. I felt the vibration of my soul, like a perfectly tuned instrument. I took a deep breath and sang a tone in a pitch that felt like it came straight from my inner spirit. It was my note, my personal pitch. I was feeling the inner music, the sound of my spirit.

If the four elements of music can bring hope to the hearts of people all over the world who have sung their way to freedom, discovered hope after genocide, awakened the spirit of creativity within, and facilitated inner peace, just think of the healing these elements can bring into your life.

I know this approach to music will encourage the healing that allows your body to dance, your heart to sing, your soul to be in harmony, your mind to rest in silence, and the inner music of your spirit to be heard and expressed in your life. But this is not just about music. It is about awakened creativity and the heart. It is about freeing your voice and spirit. It is a journey that will reverberate beyond the discovery of the medicine of music into living a harmonious life.

Welcome home.

Christine Stevens
Encinitas, CA

1

Sound Check

Have you ever gotten goose bumps from a powerful piece of music? Have you ever been moved to tears by the words of a song that express how you feel? Have you ever had a song magically play on the radio just when you need it most?

If you answered yes to these questions, you are not alone. Daniel Levitin, author of *This Is Your Brain on Music*, calls our love of music a human obsession. But music's medicine is much deeper than that. You might say that we are music. Our heartbeat is a rhythm track pulsing through our veins; our voice is the melody that resonates as we speak; our health is the harmony of our body and mind; and our breath is the silence that allows our bodies to rest. In the words of George Leonard, aikido master and pioneer of the human potential movement, "We do not make music; music makes us."[1]

When you go to a doctor's office, you get a checkup. In our journey of music for healing, we begin with a "sound check," or a quick examination of the viruses that inhibit music's medicine in our lives. I'll show you how to tune out any doubts that you are musical, and I'll share scientific evidence that confirms how innate music is within us all.

Consumers versus Creators

How have we forgotten we are all musical? How have we become music listeners more than music makers, consumers more than creators? It's often one critical statement from some authority figure that silences us. We get told we "can't carry a tune in a bucket" or that we should "just move our lips" in the choir concert.

If you've ever heard such comments, you are in good company. Sir Paul McCartney failed choir auditions twice. Luciano Pavarotti was told he needed to change his sound to be more like the "operatic greats." At the age of ten, George Gershwin was told it was too late to start studying music. Thank God they didn't stop making music. Instead they brought melodies to the hearts of music fans worldwide.

Imagine how many McCartneys have been lost because of musical criticism that silenced them and caused them to give up on their music. Imagine how many "survivors" of piano lessons shut down their musical creativity because they were told they weren't talented enough. But as we shall see, it's never too late to make your music.

Instrumentaphobia

What is going on with our musical spirit? A 2006 Gallup poll indicated that only 7.6 percent of Americans over the age of eighteen had played an instrument in the past year.[2] That's a shocking 92 percent who felt they were not musical. The poll didn't test singing, so it is possible that more of us make music than these statistics might indicate. I'm hopeful!

Three years later, a follow-up 2009 poll showed that of those who played an instrument, 95 percent started playing before age fifteen, with 72 percent starting between ages five and eleven. Only 5 percent started playing after age eighteen. There seems to be a pervasive belief that if we didn't start early on, it's too late. The poll also found that only 38 percent of homes reported that someone in the household played music; that's 62 percent of households that face music-making deprivation. When asked what would motivate these same people to play music, 95 percent of the reasons had to do with health. At some level, we intuitively know that music holds healing benefits in our lives.[3]

The same follow-up poll found that eighty-five percent of people wished that they could play an instrument. This "wish factor" cannot be extinguished. The healing benefits of music continue to call out to the soul. Guess who is among this majority? President Barack Obama, who told Barbara Walters in an interview of Ten Personal Questions that he wishes he could play a musical instrument. A separate survey in England in 2007 showed that the most common regret in older adults was not playing a musical instrument, which rated higher than not going to college, being overweight, or not taking up a sport or hobby.[4]

If music is such a universal language, why are we so tongue-tied? I call this condition *instrumentaphobia,* or the fear of playing an instrument. For many people, music has not been a positive experience; perhaps the criticism or negative experiences in choir or piano lessons had a lasting effect. Whatever the reason, this fear not only stops us from playing an instrument, it even reverberates into our creative confidence.

There is another coexisting condition, a result of suppressing our musical spirit, that I call *creative constipation.* Creativity is our birthright, an organic medicine of healing. Yet we become stifled and afraid that we are not talented enough. We strive for approval or consider ourselves untalented. We compare ourselves to the stars and feel we fall short. All these dynamics lead to a sense of withholding. Emotionally, we feel there is something inside us trying to express itself. Physically, we feel blocked, unable to access the powerful pathway of sound and music for our own well-being. Life can become boring when the spark of creative fire is not lit in the soul of our spirit.

Whatever the reason for your creative constipation, the cure is a *sonic colonic.* In this way, you can release any beliefs and insecurities you may have developed. No matter where these beliefs originated, you are the one who can remove them. Fire the inner critic and hire a coach. Make space for the call to music's medicine. Otherwise, you may never express the song of your soul that wants to be sung. As the old saying goes: don't die with the music inside you.

More Music Culture

When you do a sound check of global musical spirit, you quickly discover that the West is lagging behind the rest of the world. Much of the world is singing, dancing, and drumming with little concern about whether they have "talent" or will become "famous." Music is woven into the fabric of life in many music cultures; it is an essential medicine for creating joy, gathering community, generating hope, freeing the spirit, communing with Spirit, and educating the children.

Years ago, I visited a township school in Cape Town, South Africa, where I was invited to lead a drum circle with the students. During an initial tour of the school, I heard singing coming from a classroom. I assumed it was the music class, but when I walked in and saw the children seated on the floor singing and clapping, I was told it was a history class, where students learned history lessons through songs. Next door, I heard more music, but this time it turned out to be a math class, counting mathematical formulas through rhythms. Finally, we went into a gymnasium, and my heart lit up as more than twenty children played marimbas and drums in harmony, conducted by not one, but two music teachers.

Imagine, at a time when American educational budgets are cutting funding for the arts, in places of greater financial challenges, the music continues to live and thrive for the children and for the next generations of musically empowered souls. In many countries, funding does not determine whether there is music each day: music is a necessary aspect of the music culture of life. It is about inclusivity, community, ritual, ceremony, and the real need to co-create and keep the spirit alive.

Cultivating Seeds

Whether or not we grow up in an active music culture, there is an organic seed of music within us all. It may have dried up, not been given enough sunlight, or even been overwatered by demands on our time that drown the roots. It may have been suppressed or left untended, but a seed is always just below the surface, waiting for the nurturing conditions to activate its presence in our lives.

We learn to cultivate our musical spirit in the same way we care for a garden: with light (taking ourselves lightly) and water (being in the flow of creativity). We weed out the self-doubt and the criticism, and we fertilize the soil of creativity. Once this occurs, our lives become like a symphony, where even hardships are heard as temporary movements seeking resolution.

Here is my personal philosophical creed, a reframing of truth to replant in your belief system as we continue on this journey:

You Are Musical

The ability to be musical comes from within.
You don't have to play an instrument,
You already are an instrument.

Music is everyone's birthright.
As a child, you explored the world of sound and rhythm.
There is a musical spirit waiting to be discovered in you.
Music is not reserved for the stage.
It can be an everyday event in everyday places.
It is heard in your heartbeat, your breath, your words,
And shared in community, ceremony, prayer, and fun.
There is a reason we say we play *music.*
Music is about creativity, playfulness, and expression.
Even if you've been silenced and excluded from music making,
You are still yearning for music in your life.
You can create harmony in your life
And connect with the musical spirit that allows your soul to sing.[5]

Your Genes on Music

If you still have any doubt that we are all wired for music, science is now demonstrating just how deeply music is woven into the fabric of our DNA. This science, in turn, begins to explain the healing role that music plays in our lives. Thanks to cutting-edge research in the field of genomics, evidence shows the benefits of music for stress reduction in body, mind, and spirit, regardless of prior musical training.

A leading researcher in mind-body medicine and music is former concert pianist turned neurologist Barry Bittman, MD. His story is not uncommon among researchers of music medicine. Since Albert Einstein, who played violin, there have been many doctor-musicians and scientist-musicians who are leading the field of music medicine research today. To date, Bittman has published more than six peer-reviewed studies on music and health. He is president of the Yamaha Music and Wellness Institute and chief innovations officer of Meadville Medical Center in Meadville, Pennsylvania. For more information on these organizations, visit yamahainstitute.org and mind-body.org.

I first met Dr. Bittman at a music therapy conference in 1999. With the support of Remo, the world's largest drum company, we worked together to develop the *Health*RHYTHMS™ facilitator training program, along with Karl T. Bruhn.

Before I describe Bittman's seminal study on stress reduction and music, here is a quick background on the human genome, which contains the hereditary information encoded in our DNA/RNA sequences. Made up of an estimated 25,000 functional genes, the human genome code was cracked in June 2000 by Celera Genomics, which is now Applied Biosystems. This discovery has led to an increasing knowledge of functionality and mechanisms that directly affect our well-being and treatment of disease.

It turns out that genes respond to both internal and external conditions, which leads to the switching on or off of certain genes. How each gene responds depends on a number of factors, and, of course, each of us has a unique response to stress. Recognizing each person's individual genomic predisposition creates more specificity in the science of individualized medicine on the forefront of medical thought today.

Determined to study the deepest level of biological evidence of stress reduction through music making, Bittman designed a creative research project. First, he eliminated all subjects with prior music-making experience, ensuring that everyone was a novice (in science, this is known as exclusionary criteria). Blood samples were taken to create a baseline level of genomic activity for each subject. The blood was tested for forty-five known genomic markers of stress, which are switches that literally "turn on" biological responses associated with health challenges that range from heart disease to cancer and from diabetes to inflammatory diseases.

Next, all of the subjects went through a one-hour stress-induction phase. Participants spent one hour putting puzzles together. Much as in life, where stress is created when things don't fit together right, the puzzle pieces were designed to create stress. The pieces didn't match, and they even had pictures on both sides. In addition, subjects were frequently told, "You are doing OK, but everyone else is doing better!"

Next, researchers randomly assigned the subjects into three subgroups. The first group had to continue the stress induction with the puzzles for another hour. After the two hours, the results of their blood samples showed no change. Their stress DNA switches remained on.

The second group got to chill out; they sat around and relaxed, reading magazines and newspapers in a quiet room in comfortable chairs for another hour. This group showed a slight reversal in genomic responses, with an average of six out of forty-five genes reversed.

The third group went into a piano keyboard lab and played music together for an hour. The group followed a recreational music-making keyboard program, the Yamaha Clavinova Connection, which was designed for fun, creativity, group support, self-expression, and relaxation. Unlike in the usual structured music lesson, subjects were free to make their own music using drums and percussion sounds, emulating a drum circle, and improvising on the keyboard. When the blood samples for this group were retested, they had reversed nineteen of forty-five gene markers of stress. In other words, playing music was found to be three times more effective for reducing stress-related gene expression than simply chilling out.[6]

Future research promises even more powerful scientific evidence on a genomic level. A new study investigating the entire human genome using a similar music-research design is currently underway. Results could begin to identify the specific genes that are involved in musical expression. We are on the brink of learning so much more about the genomic basis of music and just how wired we are for music.

The Key to Music's Medicine

According to Bittman's results, as we engage in making music, we can disengage genomic triggers associated with stress. Thus, it's not only what music *does* but also what it *undoes*. There is a principle to music's medicine, an activation and deactivation pattern. It's not only what we turn on, but also what is turned off; not only what we get from music, but also what we get to let go of that is healing.

You may have noticed a similar effect in your own mood states. Notice that it's hard to be angry when you're laughing; hard to be sad when you're happy; hard to worry about the past when you're in the now. The simultaneous-state theory in psychology points to how impossible it is to be in two opposing states at the same time.

This activation/deactivation principle applies to each element of music's medicine. In rhythm, we find that drumming turns off the thinking mind and allows us to feel the primal knowledge in our bodies. In melody, we find that sounding our deep emotions transforms pain and despair and helps heal the heart. In harmony, we find that harmonizing with others turns off the "I" and activates the "we," transcending ego and filling the soul with unity. In silence, we find that quieting the mind deactivates our thinking about the past and future and allows the activation of peace and quiet.

These are not just theoretical claims. Real science documents these activation and deactivation patterns. But theory does not create change. As much as this book shows *why* we should connect with music's medicine, it is also about *how* to bring music into your life. As in most matters of growth and transformation, accessing greater creativity and self-expression is more about what we need to let go of than what we need to "get." It's about remembering and bringing forth the musical spirit within everyone.

Music is as innate as the rhythm of your heart, as close to your being as the hum of your soul, and as intrinsic as the silent space between each breath. Release any limiting beliefs you have about your own inner musical spirit and recognize that in all the elements of music, you will find a gateway into the healing benefits of sound.

2

The Medicine of Music

Music is one of the oldest forms of preventive medicine known to humanity. Long before the development of the booming music industry, music was rooted in the sacred soil of spirituality and healing. When you consider that in 2000, the money spent worldwide on music (CDs, cassettes, and vinyl records) was thirty-seven billion dollars, it may well be one of our most highly funded supplements.[1]

Music and sound are present in the language of medicine. Health means being of "sound mind and body." The Chinese word for medicine, *yao,* is derived from the word for music, *yue.*[2] But the connection is deeper than language. Medicine men and women used drumming and chanting to treat illnesses. Shamans were doctors in indigenous tribes, traveling on drumbeats to other realms to care for the soul's spiritual health. This connection of music and medicine continues today. You can see it in the researchers I've highlighted in this book—they are doctor-musicians who are contributing to the growing body of evidence-based studies that validate the intuitive wisdom of the ancients.

The term *music medicine* strengthens the value of music beyond entertainment and reconnects us to the lineage of musical healing, honoring its traditional reverence. To say "music medicine" is to move music to a place in your life beyond entertainment or distraction. Instead of tuning out, this approach allows you to use music to tune in and tune up.

Music requires no prescription. You don't need to refill it, and there are no insurance forms to fill out. Its impact is felt immediately, in what the pharmaceutical world would call a speedy uptake. I once wrote an article called "Vitamin D: Vitamin Drum," for *Natural Beauty & Health* magazine, in which I predicted that someday drums would be sold in pharmacies. I argued that music should be seen as a supplement, a daily vitamin for health and well-being. I'm still anticipating that day.

Good medicine demonstrates its effectiveness across the spectrum, from illness to wellness. In this way, music functions in treatment, prevention, health, and even personal growth. So often, people discover healing techniques or make lifestyle changes because they are facing a serious illness. But I hope people won't wait until they are sick to receive the healing benefits of music.

For many of us, the approach to health has become more holistic. It's not just about the body anymore. We are embracing a more whole-person philosophy, recognizing that we are a complex system of body, heart, soul, mind, and spirit. We are moving beyond the idea that treatment is only about our body and moving toward a growing understanding of how the mind affects our well-being. Just as we have focused on the body in relationship to how we eat, exercise, and manage stress, we now recognize the health benefits of positive thinking, hope, motivation, a sense of support, and a connection to the spiritual.

Wellness is defined as the active pursuit of health. The health-consciousness movement demonstrates that the way we live either makes us ripe for disease or creates fertile ground for wellness to take root and protect us when the flu breaks out or when stress is high. We know that stress causes negative responses in the body, such as suppressing the immune system, which increases our susceptibility to illnesses. Experts claim that an estimated 75 percent of doctor visits involve stress-related complaints.[3] Stress can inhibit the healing process, thus reducing the effectiveness of medicine and treatment. To move to greater levels of health, we must practice prevention and live a lifestyle in which well-being permeates our body, mind, and spirit.

It's important to note that music isn't a stand-alone cure. These days, there is a proliferation of products claiming to heal. But I want to be clear that the purpose of this book is to provide a guide to creating the kind of healing that comes from greater self-care, balance, wellness, and lifestyle changes.

As we orchestrate our lives as vibrant, well-tuned, and resonant human instruments, we contribute to a worldwide symphony of health and well-being. When building our repertoire of tools for healthy living, music becomes an essential practice for living a truly harmonious life. The key is in identifying your individual needs and creating your own music prescription that allows your heart to sing.

Healing through Music

Healing is a process of bringing back into life what is missing; it is a process of becoming whole. For people who have experienced a separation from music, allowing music back into their lives can invoke a surprisingly emotional healing experience.

At a health conference where I was leading a drum circle, a woman in her seventies sat in the back row with her hands crossed over her body. She did not seem very engaged; for some reason, she was resistant to joining us. Fifteen minutes into the circle, I noticed that she had picked up a small shaker and was playing along. As we continued to play, she actually moved toward the center of the circle and switched to playing a drum. She was smiling brightly and rocking out to the groove. The vibrancy was visible on her face, and she literally looked ten years younger.

After the circle, she walked up to me with tears in her eyes. She shared with me that she had a lot of stress in her life and felt constricted by the pressures of work and family obligations. The drum circle brought her relief, a way to let go for the first time. She said she never thought of herself as musical, but "something" helped her open up and discover that the less she tried to play, the better she sounded. She summed it up by saying, "You've made a loose woman of me!"

People often come up to me after their first drum circle with tears in their eyes and a look of confusion on their face. "Why am I crying?" they ask me. "I'm not sad! In fact, I feel happy." A healing experience is often accompanied by tears, which are triggered by reconnecting with something that had been missing, or what psychologists call "reunion grief."[4]

Reunion grief is a complicated concept, so I'll offer an example. Imagine you are waiting to pick up an old friend at the airport, someone you haven't seen in a long time. The moment your friend arrives, you both embrace and cry. This is rather backward, because you should cry when the person is gone, not when the person has arrived. But you often don't know what you've lost until you have it back. We cry in the embrace, in the reunion moment that holds the joy along with the recognition of the sadness that being apart had created.

Music can be like an old friend who has been away from our lives, gone from the home of our hearts. When music returns, it embraces us right back, all the way through to our bones. The healing is instantaneous.

Music's Sacred Lineage

Is it any coincidence that angels sing as well as play trumpets and harps? Hindu deities play instruments: Krishna plays the flute, and Saraswati plays the *vina*, an Indian guitar. As we move through the unfolding song of this book, I'll introduce you to deities and saints of different traditions that represent rhythm, melody, harmony, and silence. Music is at the core of many world religions. If there is indeed a pinnacle point at which all religions meet—a oneness of Spirit—music is its holy soundtrack. Sufi master Hazrat Inayat Khan said, "There will come a day when music and its philosophy will become the religion of humanity."[5]

George Harrison, guitarist of the Beatles, dove into the rich culture of spiritual wisdom and sound in India. Shrivatsa Goswami once told him, "If you read the Vedas a million times, that is equal to one recitation of the *japas* [prayer beads]. And if you do a million japas, that is equal to once making an offering of food with love to the Lord. And a million such offerings are equal to one musical offering. Then, what is superior to a musical offering? Only another musical offering. Nothing is higher. Musical offering is supreme."[6]

In music medicine, intention is the key note. A musical jingle created to sell a product has a very different intent from a mother singing a lullaby to her child at night. When music is generated as healing, devotion, or spiritual communion, it transforms the musician and the listener. The intention might be for our own self-healing or for the healing of others. You can offer music to others the way Tibetan Buddhists practice chanting, "May all beings be happy and free," or like the Lakota Native Americans, who say, "To all my relations." In this way, with clear intent and direction, your music is invoking a purpose. The seed of intention determines the outcome of the music.

The Medicine Way

According to the Lakota sacred teachings, music is medicine. Specific proto-cols surround the use of sound, in the same way that treatment protocols are used when doctors prescribe medicine. For example, songs honoring bears are not sung while bears are hibernating in the winter. Lakota ceremonies begin with welcoming songs and end with gratitude songs. Tobacco is placed as an offering on the drum before the drum is played. The reverence for the "song medicine" and the "drum medicine" defines the healing power of music in Lakota and other indigenous traditions. When used this way, the term *medicine* refers to something that gives us energy for body, mind, and spirit. As Lakota medicine man Peter Catches says, "Food is our number one medicine, because we are sustained by it and we gain strength from it; we are happy when we are well fed and glad to be alive. It makes us strong and happy."[7] Music can be as nourishing as food, a medicine for the soul.

In more than a decade of doing ceremonies with both the Lakota Nation and the Women's Way Long Dance, I often heard people say, "That's your medicine," referring to an individual's particular talent or the healing quality that person possessed. This medicine could be the leadership gift of the chief or facilitator or the way someone knows how to care for a child. In fact, elders in the community recognize and call out the talents in others before the individuals themselves are even aware of those talents.

In both groups, I was told many times that music is my medicine. This idea resonated deeply within me, yet I had no idea how profoundly these words would affect my life. As a board-certified music therapist, it gave me a less clinical way to state what I felt my gift was: I was not just playing my music; I was also bringing forth the music in others.

The Medicine Wheel

In the words of Lakota Chief Black Elk, "Birds make their nests in circles; the circle is the sun and moon and all round things in the natural world. The circle is an endless creation."[8]

For the Lakota and other indigenous people, the circle forms the basis of the medicine wheel. Initially I was introduced to this cosmology while spending a year learning the four directions of the medicine wheel with my teacher Kathy Hull. This medicine wheel is based upon cultural anthropolo-gist Angeles Arrien's book *The Four-Fold Way*. I had no idea the impact the medicine wheel would have on my life and on my spiritual understanding. It shifted me from my Methodist upbringing, which had taught me that God was above and I was below, to a sense of the sacred all around and within me.

To give you a basic picture of how the medicine wheel works, here is a simple explanation for this large concept: The circle of the medicine wheel contains four sections, which represent the four cardinal directions—east, west, north, and south. When taken separately, each direction has teachings, power animals, and a representative color. The east brings the medicine of the new day, the time of childhood, and the season of spring. The south brings the medicine of coyote (the trickster), the time of adolescence, and the season of summer. The west brings the time of dusk, the setting sun, the time of adulthood, and the season of autumn. Finally, the north brings the medicine of owl (wisdom), the time of elderhood, and the season of winter. The specifics that each direction represents vary by tribe, but the directions are universal, reflecting nature and the planet.

The medicine wheel is also multidimensional. In addition to the four directions, there is the presence above in Father Sky and below in Mother Earth. Like any circle, there is also a point at the center where everything meets in the middle. The center is in the heart of every person; it is the indwelling of Spirit. The center is within you.

The sacredness of the circle and the four directions also appears in other world traditions. You see it in the neopagan, earth-based traditions, in which the four directions relate to the four elements of earth, air, fire, and water. In Tibetan Buddhism, the circle is a mandala with four directions that are associated with specific seed sounds, representing teachings and depicted with different colors. Psychiatrist Carl Jung devoted much of his life to using mandalas as a tool for exploring deeper states of consciousness, creating universal archetypes of healing. Angeles Arrien identified four archetypes—warrior, teacher, visionary, and healer—which aligned with each direction in the circle cosmologies of world traditions. Some say the four gospels in the Bible and the four archangels further echo this theme.

A Hoop of Harmony

For me, the medicine wheel was an obvious parallel with music. Music is its own medicine wheel, a circle of sound that holds many analogies with the cycles of nature and life. There are twelve chromatic notes in the scale, like the twelve months of the year. The drum is a circle, and the drum circle is set up in its natural healing shape. In the music of tabla drumming from India, rhythms are even notated on a rhythm clock in cycles of twelve or sixteen. Even deeper than that, harmonic motion in music moves in a circle called the *circle of fifths* or the *music wheel*. In addition, the sacred sense of four is evident when we sing in four-part harmony.

The four directions in the medicine wheel relate to the four elements of music: rhythm, melody, harmony, and silence. The fifth element is the center, the direction that is within you. This model also mirrors the seasons of life. Rhythm is a natural starting point in the direction of the east, the position of sunrise, where life begins with a pulse and the playfulness of childhood. Traveling clockwise around the circle, melody comes next as the developing song of our individual identity, the season of adolescence. Harmony brings us into relationships, maturing us in the season of adulthood, the direction of the west. Silence brings completion to the circle and represents the quiet wisdom of the season of elderhood, the direction of the north. The inner music represents the timeless season of *now* we live in our entire lives.

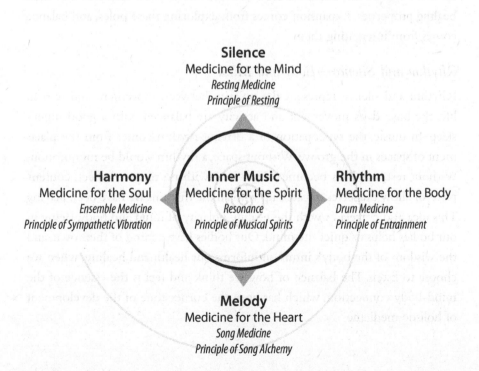

Silence
Medicine for the Mind
Resting Medicine
Principle of Resting

Harmony
Medicine for the Soul
Ensemble Medicine
Principle of Sympathetic Vibration

Inner Music
Medicine for the Spirit
Resonance
Principle of Musical Spirits

Rhythm
Medicine for the Body
Drum Medicine
Principle of Entrainment

Melody
Medicine for the Heart
Song Medicine
Principle of Song Alchemy

This model is not only a two-dimensional wheel, but it is also a spiral of sound. As we develop our musical spirit, we spiral through these elements in cycles of growth. The inner music is expressed and shared as we take part in orchestrating change in the world. We become living examples of peace and harmony.

The circular model is a picture of wholeness and a path to personal healing. Each element of music has gifts for our emotional, biological, social, and spiritual health. We usually talk about our self as being composed of mind, body, and spirit, but I also add heart and soul.

Key principles associated with each element further extend the benefits of music into our lives. They bring teachings and medicine. Drum medicine, song medicine, ensemble medicine, and resting medicine are the gifts of the four main elements of music. Going within to the center of the circle, we find the inner music, whose medicine is resonance.

Polarity and Balance

Polarities are inherent in the circle. Polarity is the pull between opposites, such as masculine and feminine, sun and moon, positive and negative. Similarly, in music's medicine, polarities exist between the musical elements and their healing properties. Expansion comes from exploring these poles, and balance comes from integrating them.

Rhythm and Silence—Body and Mind

Rhythm and silence represent the polarity between movement and rest. In life, the busy day's movement and activity are balanced with a good night's sleep. In music, the syncopation of a driving rhythm comes from the placement of spaces in the groove. Without space, a rhythm would be monotonous. Without rest, our lives become a busy beat with no time to reflect, contemplate, or allow ourselves to catch up with all the rhythms we have been playing. This idea also correlates with the healing polarity of mind and body. Being in our bodies helps us quiet the mind. Our bodies have a mind of their own, and the wisdom of the body's intuition informs our health and healing, when we choose to listen. The balance of how we think and feel is the essence of the mind-body connection, which has been the cornerstone of the development of holistic medicine.

Melody and Harmony—Heart and Soul

Melody and harmony represent the polarity between individuality and interconnectedness. In music, melody is the solo line, whereas harmony is the ensemble. Melody is "I"; harmony is "we." Melody is singular; harmony is collective. Within this polarity, we balance being true to our authentic voice while living in harmony with the world around us, calibrated and in concert. This is also the healing polarity of heart and soul. Like the body, the heart is temporary, but the soul is eternal. The heart carries us to our individual passion, while the soul carries us to our purpose in serving community.

Inner Music and Outer Music—Being and Doing

The inner and outer music represent the polarity between being and doing. The inner music is internal, while the use of music for orchestrating change is external. With inner music, we are tuning our human instrument, and with outer music, we are tuning in to the growing movement of creating music for global peace and for healing in the world. We balance our personal needs with our desire to serve the world with our gifts. Healers often run the risk of becoming depleted by overgiving without staying attuned to their inner needs and their own practice of self-care. We cannot give when we are depleted. But when we are inwardly satisfied, we become available to be an offering to the sound healing of the world.

Ocean of Sound

How does music's medicine relate to our personal healing? I like to use the metaphor of the ocean. The ocean contains buoyancy, rhythm, currents, and the ebb and flow of the tides coming in and going out. Similarly, music creates a bidirectional current of healing that flows like the ocean tides, moving into us as we consciously listen and moving out through us as we express ourselves in sound. We invoke and evoke, receive and express music's medicine. It's as natural as breathing; listening to music is the inhale, while expressing sound is the exhale. In music medicine, both directions create healing opportunities, which scientific studies have shown to be effective.

Current becomes cyclical in sound. When you express music, you simultaneously listen. The flow becomes a circuit of sound that is amplified when you make music with others. Participating in the circuitry of sound is the way we support each other and build on the energy together. Research studies show that group music-making experiences often show greater benefits than do solo experiences. In the ping-pong energetic flow of musical dialogue, the sound moves in waves that crest and settle. Every jam session is its own topography.

Floating in this powerful energy of music's medicine requires a paradigm change. Don't think of music as something you have to attain; rather, think of it as something that wants to flow through you.

The following poetic Sutra 60, from the *Vijnana Bhairava Tantra* that dates back to 800 CE, is translated from the original Sanskrit by Dr. Lorin Roche in *The Radiance Sutras*. It explains our natural connection to the ocean of sound:

> *Beloved, listen.*
> *The ocean of sound is inviting you*
> *Into its spacious embrace,*
> *Calling you home.*
> *Find that exuberant vibration*
> *Rising new in every moment,*
> *Humming in your secret places,*
> *Resounding through the channels of delight.*
> *Know you are flooded by it always.*
> *Float with the sound,*
> *Melt with it into divine silence.*
> *The sacred power of space will carry you*
> *Into the dancing radiant emptiness*
> *That is the source of all.* [9]

Whether we are consciously listening to music or we are expressing it, the healing lies in being open to receive and willing to express.

Receiving Music's Medicine—Conscious Listening

An old Biblical story serves as an early case study of musical healing through listening. The story goes that King Saul had become depressed and felt that the spirit of the Lord had left him. You might say he was facing a dark night of the soul. Desperate to restore King Saul's health, his servants suggested music. They went out to find David, a known warrior and also a harpist, who was tending to his sheep. David came to the palace to play for the king. According to the story, when the music started, Saul immediately felt better.

How much of this healing was David's playing, and how much was Saul's openness to receive the music? No matter how good the music, Saul could not have been healed without his spirit being open to receive David's harp playing. When we hear live music, we are offered a kinesthetic and vibrational experience. Saul allowed the music into the wounded places of his soul, seeking to be reconnected to Spirit.

The gateway is within us as receivers. How open we are to music determines how much of its medicinal effect we will receive. When we consciously listen with our whole being, we deeply receive, allowing music to pour into our veins, touch our hearts and souls, and move us at our core. We can feel it in our bones.

Conscious versus Unconscious Listening

Music piped into elevators, grocery stores, and lobbies causes us to become conditioned to "background" music. But when we listen consciously, we bring the background to the foreground and move from hearing to listening. Healing music is filled with nutrition. However, when we are unconscious or take music for granted, it does nothing for our deep need to be fed. We may be hungry, but music's nutritional value cannot be absorbed without our participation to ingest and digest its supplement value.

When we close our eyes, sound changes. Listening to music through headphones is different from listening through earbuds. Attending a concert or listening to live music is different from hearing recorded music. The secret to achieving the most from music is in how we listen. If we sit still, we can feel the rhythm move us. When we place a hand on our hearts, we direct the current of music there. In this way, we become instruments of our own healing.

Your Inner DJ

Can you think of a time when hearing a song lifted your mood, helped you through a hard time, or brought healing into your life? When it comes to music, we all have distinct preferences, and it turns out that the music we love is a key to its healing benefits.

A study from Glasgow Caledonian University in Scotland compared the effect of three different kinds of music on reducing pain for nearly sixty subjects. Participants listened to one of three types of recorded music: music they chose (listener preference), music specifically designed for relaxation, or white noise. The effectiveness of the music was tested for its power to reduce the perception of pain and provide a sense of control. Not surprisingly, the greatest benefit in both pain reduction and perceived sense of control came with a listener's preferred music.[10]

Music's medicine is individualized, determined by your unique sense of connection to the music that draws you in. What sound is music to your ears? There's a reason certain music resonates with you. The music you like—classical, rock, bluegrass, folk, hip-hop, jazz, and so on—facilitates the healing response. I call it your "inner DJ."

Trust the music you love. Seek it out when you need it most. Listen for what music moves you, and then store that music in the vitamin closet of your iPod.

The Goose Bump Effect

Scientific evidence can help explain why listening to our favorite music gives us goose bumps (the medical term is *piloerection*). A seminal study from the Addiction Research Foundation examined the thrill response elicited by listening to music. Avram Goldstein, MD, of Stanford University designed an experiment to study the neurobiological-emotional process of how music creates a natural high.

Goldstein first asked college-age subjects to describe the sensation of thrills they felt when listening to music. You may relate to the results: most subjects identified the thrill as originating in the upper spine and the back of the neck. Medium thrills lasted about one to five seconds, whereas more intense thrills lasted longer and actually spread throughout the body, radiating upward to the head and face, down the spine, into the chest, and down through the thighs and legs. That's a pretty intense physiological reaction to sound.

Second, Goldstein compared listening to music with other experiences that could elicit thrills. Surprisingly, 96 percent of the participants agreed that the number one stimuli that created thrills was a musical passage. Music outperformed many things we generally think of as thrilling, including physical contact with another person, sexual activity, watching a favorite sports team win, or moments of inspiration.

Once he had a clearer understanding of the basis of this natural arousal from music, Goldstein had subjects sit in a dark room and listen to their chosen music through headphones, creating the conditions that amplify the powerful effect of listening to music. The subjects were asked to indicate their thrill sensations in terms of frequency, duration, and intensity.

Results indicated that thrill responses often matched the contour of the music, especially when there was a surprise or a sudden change in the familiar. On a neurochemical level, Goldstein discovered that musical thrills stimulated the release of opioid peptides, which are endorphins that connect to the brain's limbic emotional area and that trigger the neurophysiological chemistry of a natural high. Blocking these receptors with the opioid inhibitor naloxone caused the thrills to decrease while listening to the same music, confirming this neurological connection.[11]

Expressing Music's Medicine—Creative Freedom

When we express music, we release emotions and tension; we give voice to feelings for which words alone cannot suffice. The music may be the sound of wailing that releases deep grief or the sound of a mother singing a lullaby to her child. Often it's the sounding of deep trauma that happened at a preverbal time in a child's life. Even if we don't know what it means, musical expression allows healing and also provides a vehicle for each person's unique voice to be shared.

We all have the capacity for musical expression. The most immediate access to musical expression comes through drumming and singing, probably because these are our biological instruments—the drum of our hearts and the song of our voice.

Benefits of Making Music

In two separate studies, which I'll cover in more depth later in this book, researchers compared active music making (in the form of drumming and singing) with music listening. In a study by Bittman, subjects who drummed in a drum circle designed for wellness were compared with another group of subjects who only listened to drum music.[12] All subjects in the study were complete novices, eliminating the effect of prior musical training that would skew results. By screening out experienced drummers, the study clearly demonstrated that we all have the capacity to express ourselves creatively through rhythm for health benefits. Results showed that active drumming resulted in greater biological changes. This result was echoed in Gunter

Kreutz's study on singing, which looked at biological markers of immune function in addition to emotional states.[13] In both studies, music making was shown to elicit greater changes in subjects' immune function, mood improvement, and morale boosting, as compared with listening.

At least three factors explain the results:

1. *Exercise.* Active music making engages us physically. It is a form of exercise. When we sing, we breathe deeply and increase our lung capacity. When we drum, we use our upper body muscles and cardiovascular system, and we get an even greater workout by moving to the beat.

2. *Self-expression.* Personal expression is healing. It's a long-demonstrated principle that withholding emotions leads to stress and medical problems. Music making allows expression and release, especially when we make up our own music in the rich freedom of being given permission to feel our way into our own sound, voice, and rhythm.

3. *Group support.* When making music together in a way that is filled with permission, support, and camaraderie, the result is healing. The key is the design of the music-making experience—that is, putting people at ease with the music-making process instead of stressing them out with demands of performance. Feeling supported by others and experiencing the sense of harmony and togetherness inherent in actually making music together is key to music's healing benefits.

This is not to say that music making should replace music listening or that spending individual time in sound won't help your biology. It's not a question of either-or. Research demonstrates that the healing effects of making music have to do with our attitude toward the experience—the "how" and the "why" and even the "with whom" we make music.

Dive In

The ocean of sound awaits your discovery. It is much simpler than you can imagine. It is a journey born of releasing any doubts that you are musical and realizing that you can access the healing benefits of music for body, mind, spirit, heart, and soul.

Each element of music is a gateway, a portal into the core of music's medicine. Each chapter comprises four sections: the art, science, spirit, and medicine of each element of music. First, the art inspires greater knowledge of the rich beauty and metaphors inherent in each distinct element of music. It also features a key principle that explains each element's power, as well as the shadow side of that power. Second, scientific evidence provides deeper explanations of each element of music and how it improves our health and well-being. Third, spiritual wisdom from many traditions describes the inspiration and lineage of the sacred use of music. Lastly, the medicine of each music element is a gift of discovery for your personal healing. Rhythm brings drum medicine, melody brings song medicine, harmony brings ensemble medicine, silence brings resting medicine, and the inner music brings the resonance of your unique spirit.

The guided practices in this book give you practical, fun, enjoyable, and often profound ways to bring music's healing into your life and the lives of the people you serve. Each section includes practices for conscious listening to and expressing of music, allowing you to swim in the ocean of sound and discover what most resonates with you based upon your own needs. Specifically designed music playlists (streaming at SoundsTrue.com/ MusicMedicine) accompany the practices. You can listen to specific tracks that accompany a practice, enjoy the music while reading, or listen to the entire playlist any time you want to bring the healing energy of music into your life. This is why I like to say that this is a book that *sings.*

At the end of this book, there is a guide for using music in personal and professional development. For self-care, there are easy steps to assess your needs and implement these teachings and techniques into your life. For music teachers, coaches, healing arts practitioners, therapists, life coaches, and teambuilding facilitators, there are recommended tools based on the guided practices that can easily be incorporated into your work. There are also questions for book club leaders, developed with the advice of my best friend, Zena Elliot, an avid reader and discussion leader. For ongoing ideas, videos, updated research, and interactive sharing opportunities, visit ubdrumcircles.com/musicmedicine.

Let the journey begin.

3

Rhythm: Medicine for the Body

This is the story of how we begin to remember
This is the powerful pulsing of blood in the veins
After the dream of falling and calling your name out
These are the roots of the rhythm and
The roots of the rhythm remain.

—PAUL SIMON, "UNDER AFRICAN SKIES," *GRACELAND*

There is a rhythm that unites us all; a pulse of humanity that is healing. Rhythm calls the body to dance and the tribe to gather. The unstoppable drum plays, and the dance goes on.

A few years ago, I was invited to lead drum circles for healing with a group of Sudanese refugees known as the Lost Boys and Lost Girls. The story of their exodus is famous. Mostly from Dinka and Nuer ethnic groups, more than twenty thousand boys and girls were orphaned during the Second Sudanese Civil War. After witnessing the brutal killing of their parents, they walked more than one thousand miles across three countries to reach refugee camps in Ethiopia and Kenya. A large population ended up in Phoenix, Arizona, where a cultural center was created for them. The center then contacted me, seeking innovative ways to treat their trauma, adjustment disorders, and resulting addiction problems. The roots of rhythm in Sudan made drumming a perfect fit for healing and for community building as they worked to establish their lives in America.

The first day of the training began with a drum-circle demonstration, which was followed by teaching the students how to lead the drum circle. We showed them how drumming could be used for expression of emotions, release, and community building. They showed us their cultural rhythms from the rich roots of rhythm in southern Sudan.

By the afternoon of the first day, word had spread that we were there, and before we knew it, local Sudanese people from the church and extended family started to arrive for the afternoon session. The room kept filling up, and the rhythms, chants, and dances kept coming. Even though more than sixty-five languages are spoken in southern Sudan, and each separate tribal group has its own rhythms, songs, and dances, we were witnessing a collaborative eruption of healing and community bonding.

For the next two hours, we all joined in the dancing and drumming of African heritage. As the rhythm finally quieted down, we came together as one in a healing moment. We stood in a circle as each person shared what he or she had received from the day. One man spoke of his longing for home, while also offering his gratitude for being given a new life. Others said they felt the sense of community and family that was created that day. But it was the comment from one young man that most moved my heart. He simply said, "I have not danced in eight years, not since I arrived in America. In the rhythms, I can go back home. Music can take you home."

Life Is a Dance

We are incubated in rhythm. Our mother's heartbeat is the soundtrack of our first concert in the womb. Rhythm reaches the inner heartbeat that is the drum within us all, the memory of the sound from a time before birth. Rhythm is everyone's homeland.

Rhythm is defined as the elements of music pertaining to forward motion. Rhythm moves us forward in life when we face challenges or feel stuck. Rhythm helps us move into a new stage. We call it our "mojo"—the movement of growth, transformation, and energy. Our bodies become alive in the beat of a good groove, energized in the spirit of rhythm, and grounded in the heartbeat of Mother Earth.

Our expressions reflect the significance of rhythm in our lives. A good mood is said to be upbeat. We say we have to "get our groove back" or "dance to the beat of our own drum." When we work together well, we are "in sync," and we say, "Timing is everything."

The body is a powerful rhythmic convergence of multiple beats working together in the groove of life. We breathe, talk, eat, chew, sleep, wake, and move to a rhythm. We are walking, talking, ticking, tocking polyrhythms of multiple beats. We embody rhythm in the pulmonary rhythm of breathing, the cardio rhythm of the heartbeat, and the circadian rhythm of sleeping and waking. Brain rhythms are measured in electroencephalogram (EEG) patterns, neural rhythms occur in firing patterns, and women's hormonal rhythms follow their menstrual cycles.

We must marvel at the rhythmicity of the human body and recognize why our bodies are so driven by rhythm. Perhaps these inner rhythms are why we all have an innate sense of timing in our bodies. We may experience this timing when we wake up just before the alarm clock goes off. This rhythm is the primal basis of our biorhythmic human nature—our rhythmical intuition—and is further evidence of our body's innate musical knowledge.

The medicine of rhythm is as much what it *undoes* as what it *does*. Rhythm is a healing force that takes us out of our minds and into our bodies, tuning out cerebral thought and activating instinctive primal knowledge. We can become overthinkers, obsessing about the details of our lives and listening to the endless chatter of self-critique and wandering mental musings. Samuel Beckett said, "Dance first and think afterward. . . . It's the natural order."[1] We can get lost in the past or future, but rhythm takes us to the beat of the now, welcoming us into the rich aliveness of every new moment.

Movement Deficit Disorder

As society becomes more removed from the rhythms of the natural world, our bodies suffer. Movement is down, and obesity is up. A lethargic lifestyle replaces physical labor. Watching television replaces the dance of joy. According to recent data from the American Heart Association, the percentage of youth ages eighteen and under who do no physical activity is shockingly high.[2] In 2007, thirty percent of girls and seventeen percent of boys polled in grades nine through twelve reported that they had not done even sixty minutes of moderate to vigorous physical activity once in the previous week.[3] This rising sedentary rhythm affects adults as well, with a shocking thirty-six percent of adults reporting no vigorous activity in the past week.

Rhythm too often becomes the monotonous beat of typing on keypads instead of joyous drumming and dancing. We sit at computers more than ever, creating an increasingly inactive lifestyle. It's no wonder that more than one-third (at least thirty-four percent) of adults in the United States are obese. In children, the numbers are alarming: thirty-two percent of children aged two to nine are obese, while another sixteen percent are overweight, making a total of forty-eight percent already facing the challenges of weight problems that lead to diseases ranging from diabetes to heart conditions.[4]

How do we remedy these conditions and restore the body's health that is crucial to our well-being? The answer lies in activating the rhythms of life, engaging more fully with the joy of being in rhythm—the music medicine of being alive.

The Art of Rhythm

Rhythm literally is the pulse, the life force, of music's medicine. Rhythm organizes time and sets the beat that allows all the other elements of music to coexist. Pulse, duration, and tempo are aspects of rhythm that move music through its dynamics of fast, slow, and everything in between. But the best place to discover the artistry of the beat is within the body. Rhythm is all about feeling.

Years ago, when I was studying music therapy at Michigan State University, I nearly failed the required percussion class. I found it hard to coordinate the drumsticks to play drum rolls and read the music. Thanks to a private drum tutor, I did pass, but the class left me feeling that I was rhythmically challenged. Years later, I attended my first drum circle in upstate New York. I remember putting my hands on conga drums for the first time. It was a whole different connection to rhythm—it was not defined by notes on a page, but by my own beat. As people danced freely in the center of the circle, I noticed I couldn't hold still. My feet were tapping and my hips were rocking, even as I drummed. Three hours went by in an instant, and I was hooked. I had fallen into the power of percussion and the art of rhythm.

Later that year, I took a *djembe* hand-drumming class with a visiting African teacher. The whole first hour was devoted to dancing and movement games. According to the teacher's tradition, you first learn to move before you learn to drum; the body and the beat were inseparable. What a contrast to my experience in college: trying to learn to read percussion music, counting the beats in my head, and struggling to transfer the groove to the drumsticks. Our African drum teacher showed me how to trust the rhythm in my body, which led to better drumming.

Four Rhythms of Life

We know rhythm from our bodies, and rhythm helps us be reconnected to our body's wisdom. The medicine goes both ways. We all have rhythm within us. This rhythm is so natural that we hardly notice the drum of who we are. The following are just a few examples of four rhythms we know from being alive that define the movement of life.

1. *Heartbeat.* The heartbeat rhythm is primal—the mother of all rhythms and the rhythm we first heard inside our mother's womb. The groove of life ranges from a resting heart rate of seventy-two beats a minute, or *adagio,* which literally means "at ease," to *andante,* or moderate, like a walking pace. When you question your own innate rhythmical sense, just remember this inner beat pulsing within you always. If you are alive, you've got rhythm.

2. *Breathing.* The beat of breathing is a natural balanced pattern of inhale and exhale. Breathing is the rhythm of life that gives the body the chance to receive and release. How we breathe creates great impact on our health, and our breath is a barometer of our state of being. Relax, and we breathe more deeply. Under stress, our breath becomes shallow. Become aware of this breathing rhythm, and you will be more present and connected to your body.

3. *Walking.* Walking is a two-beat pattern, a double beat, which in music is called "duple meter." The walking beat has a masculine energy, like marching forward, feeling a sense of linear movement, straight ahead. Military chants are formed to this rhythm, but so are samba grooves in Brazilian street parades. In the walking beat, we learn the subtle contrast between downbeat and upbeat. In the downbeat, we feel a sense of grounding, like steps walking on the earth. In the upbeat, we feel lifted in the magical space between each pulse. *(Listen to tracks 9 and 10 from the rhythm playlist at the end of this chapter.)*

4. *Rocking*. Rocking back and forth or swaying creates a soothing, more feminine groove. We all know it from the motion of being rocked as babies. Rocking inspires the hips to move in the sensuality and circularity of undulating motions. Rocking is a triple meter or three-beat pattern. We hear this rhythm in many world beats, from Africa to Brazil, and in cultures that live in more connection to the feminine energy of Mother Earth. *(Listen to tracks 2 and 7 from the rhythm playlist.)*

Polyrhythm

Life's rhythms do not exist separately; they are woven together in a multitasking groove of polyrhythm, a word that means "many rhythms." The art of polyrhythm is felt in the way two different rhythms coexist and ultimately come together. Even in a composition of seemingly different beats, there is periodic alignment, much like with our body rhythms. The duple meter of the walking beat and the triple meter of the rocking beat line up every twelfth beat, creating a reverberating "one" where the pulse is felt the strongest. An underlying consistent pulse ties it all together.

The Groove—The Pocket of Life

The groove in music is the feeling that calls our bodies to dance easily and effortlessly. It's the underlying essence of the rhythmical force that holds music together. Good drummers learn to establish the groove and then fall into it, maintaining a consistent energy. The groove is a pathway, a portal, a secret spot that drummers call "the pocket," a place of rhythmic alignment where playing becomes effortless.

Being in the groove also happens in life when we create the groove that is our essence; it's our way of moving through life, sharing our gifts, growing, and dancing. We can tell when we're in the groove. Life lines up, and we feel a sense of being carried by the rhythm of our daily movements and interactions. Gradually we learn to trust the groove and take risks; and we do so more and more effortlessly. Life becomes a dance to the beat of our own drum, building the "mojo" upon every beat of our life as we step forward, sometimes in uncharted compositions orchestrated by our own heartbeat.

Tune in to your own life's groove and notice the tempo changes. Be courageous and share the beat of your own heart. Notice how you create the pocket of life—the place where your gifts line up with the opportunity to serve, grow, and create.

Synchronicity

When rhythms line up in life's magical moments of perfect timing in an unplanned way, it is synchronicity. Synchronicity is an awareness of the rhythm of seemingly coincidental events occurring in perfect timing. Synchronicity in life's magical moments reflects a perfect timing beyond our own planning. *Chronos,* the root of *synchronicity,* literally means "timing." When we recognize these synchronicities, we experience an even greater groove of life. It seems that things come together beyond our own personal efforts. Perhaps you have had an intuition to call a friend just at the moment she needs your support. Or maybe you are in the right place at the right time for a new career opportunity. When this happens, you are playing your life like a drummer in the pocket, the groove—and this is your rhythm.

When we live according to our life's purpose, synchronicity grows. The key to this is to practice recognizing synchronicity, like a drummer listening for moments when the beats align perfectly, effortlessly. Then we can receive the magic and trust the effortless unfolding of our rhythm.

Think of a time when you experienced synchronicity in your life that was an amazing moment. Be aware of this rhythm in your life.

The Principle of Rhythm—Entrainment

Do you ever experience a feeling of being in sync with someone, a sense of shared groove that carries you easily? Do you ever notice how people walking down the street naturally fall in step with one another without being aware of it? These phenomena are actually part of a principle of physics called *entrainment,* which means the synchronizing of separate rhythms.

Scientist Christian Huygens is attributed with the discovery of entrainment in 1656, when he observed how pendulums naturally fall in sync over time. According to entrainment, a dominant oscillator will draw surrounding rhythms into its sway, causing things ultimately to move together in concert. Our bodies are wired for entrainment as well. Our circadian rhythms of sleeping and waking are entrained by light; we feel sleepy in the dark of night and awaken to the rays of sunlight. Women's menstrual cycles often entrain to lunar cycles and to each other.

Evidence of this principle is also at play in nature. If you've ever watched the movie *Winged Migration* or simply been mesmerized by the way birds fly together, you've witnessed the musical tailwind of rhythm. By flapping their wings in perfect succession, migrating birds use up to 70 percent less effort compared with individual flight. The beating of wings in this shared groove sustains the birds' journey for thousands of miles. Just think what you could do with 70 percent more energy. The lesson is profound. Moving in rhythm together is the easiest way to travel the distance.

The Shadow Side of Rhythm

Entrainment has its challenges as well. We can underestimate the power of rhythm and the potential for being pulled into something that we cannot get out of. If you've ever gone into the workplace and felt pulled into the negative energy of coworkers' complaining, you have experienced a sense of entrainment. The danger is in losing your own beat by getting pulled into a stagnant rhythm. The medicine of rhythm helps recalibrate our beat, restore and renew our sense of self, and find that inner beat that only we can play.

We can also get stuck in a rhythm and find it hard to change. Strong grooves are tough to break. Changing patterns and habits in life is like going against a strong rhythm. We can get stuck in the groove of an argument or get lost in a groove that's not healthy. As in music, we need a moment of silence to clear the history of the past rhythm and create a new beat. This is how rhythm and silence, as polarities in music's medicine wheel, support one another.

Then there are the tempo changes. When the tempo varies, in both music and in life, it's often more challenging to slow down *(ritardando)* than it is to speed up *(accelerando)*. Does this sound familiar? The tempo often speeds up to create the rising of energy and slows down to create a settling peacefulness that invites us inward. Tempo changes affect the dance, the rhythm, and our lives on a daily basis. The challenge to the shadow side of rhythm is recognizing entrainment, groove locking, and tempo changes and empowering ourselves to be the orchestrators of our own new beat.

The Science of Rhythm

From the simple act of walking to the creative beauty of dance, rhythm speaks to our bodies and expresses our innate groove. It is a deep biological, neurological pathway that we can access for healing, growth, and development.

Rhythm and Rehabilitation

The Center for Biomedical Research in Music at Colorado State University, run by Michael Thaut, PhD, has made great strides in the research of entrainment. This is also where I received my master's degree. For more information on the center, visit colostate.edu/dept/cbrm.

Thaut's team has been creating a neurological model of music therapy built upon entrainment mechanisms that link rhythm with the body's natural rhythmicity. They have found that rhythm can stimulate damaged areas of the brain that are otherwise unreachable. Their original area of research was working with walking, or gait. They found that by turning on a metronome that beats to a tempo that matches the subjects' normal walking patterns, the gait of the subjects improved in three areas—cadence, velocity, and stride length. This finding was then applied successfully to patients going through physical therapy.

In a seminal study, Thaut's team showed that rhythm significantly and immediately improved the walking patterns of patients with Parkinson's disease, who typically suffer from shuffling and uneven walking patterns and who, in extreme cases, sometimes become frozen and unable to move. After taking a baseline of the subjects' walking tempo, the team provided music with a matched beat. Immediately, the music gave the patients a better sense of timing, and by walking to the music, they improved their gait. A breakthrough came when the researchers increased the rhythm by 10 percent; in response, the patients' walking naturally sped up, without any extensive training or effort. The presence of the beat helped improve the patients' stride length, distance, and walking tempo.[5] The team named this therapeutic intervention rhythmic auditory stimulation (RAS).

While I was at Colorado State University, I saw live demonstrations of this study. It was like watching miracles happen. Without music playing, patients were clumsy and unbalanced as they walked across the room in silence. But once the rhythm of the music started to play, there was an immediate sense of ease and balance, a sustained flow and grace as they walked to the beat. Thaut's team created a simpler, more natural, and definitely more enjoyable tune for physical rehabilitation. By giving patients a soundtrack to practice with at home, the researchers helped patients internalize the music, giving them a song to hum in their minds to activate movement when their bodies became frozen.

Thaut's team had similarly successful results when they tested RAS on other populations with brain disorders who had suffered a stroke or who had cerebral palsy. Their findings led to an interesting question as to where specifically in the brain entrainment happens. Because Parkinson's disease damages higher cerebral areas, Thaut began to explore the deeper aspects of the neurology of the lower brain areas—specifically, the cerebellum. His team found that this ancient "reptilian" brain area was key to entrainment. When patients heard the rhythm, a subconscious effect occurred. The patients did not have to think; they had the natural impulse to move to the beat.[6] You might say that rhythm goes without thinking.

Thaut's team further identified how rhythm helps the body's physiology organize to the timing cue of rhythm, synchronizing the many complex sub-aspects involved in movement. The beat improves coordination by creating a rhythm target. The body knows intuitively how to make everything line up, beyond our ability to "think" it out. Without rhythm, the body faced fatigue due to overexertion. With rhythm, the body knew when to turn on bursts of effort and when to turn it off. The pattern of effort and rest is our best use of physical resources, a natural process felt best through rhythm.

Extending Thaut's demonstration of lower brain areas involved in entrainment, a music therapy research team tested group drumming with Alzheimer's patients. Alzheimer's disease is an organic brain disease that causes damage in the higher brain areas, where short-term memory and cognitive tasks are processed. Despite memory loss and confusion, patients not only entrained in drumming, they even improved over time. This is due in part to the entrainment centers in the undamaged lower brain—the cerebellum. Remarkably, week after week, the patients' drumming improved. Even with a brain disease affecting memory, the patients were learning. Group drumming gave the isolated patients a social experience, a voice of self-expression, and a sense of accomplishment and control. These are very healing experiences needed in the care of our elderly in senior centers.[7]

Beating Stress

Cutting-edge research in psychoneuroimmunology and mind-body medicine shows that rhythm can enhance the immune system on a cellular level. For the first time, scientific research has validated why rhythm is one of the oldest tools of music medicine, one that has withstood the test of time.

In 2000, Barry Bittman, MD, performed the first biological research study on the impact of group drumming on the immune system. All the subjects in the experiment were healthy individuals who had no prior musical or drumming experience. The experiment compared three groups: a resting control group that sat and read magazines, a listening group that just listened to drumming music, and a drum-circle experience in which subjects played rhythms together led by a drum-circle facilitator. Blood samples were taken before and after the one-hour experiment to test key indicators of the immune system, our body's natural defense system against disease and virally infected cells. These blood tests included tests for dehydroepiandrosterone (DHEA), cortisol, natural killer (NK) cell activity, and other cytokines that are considered orchestrators of the immune system.

However, not all experiments go as planned. After the first drum-circle test, Bittman found no significant changes in the experimental group compared with the control group. His research team then tried different approaches to drumming, using less talking or leading the drumming by a local shaman, but still no significant results occurred. It's important to note that some subjects reported feeling better or having fun, but it did not change their biology. Finally, it became apparent that the subjects were actually intimidated by drumming. Performance anxiety and a fear of making a mistake or losing the beat were causing their stress to rise. This anxiety was driving biology in the wrong direction.

Working with an interdisciplinary team, Bittman developed a friendlier approach to the act of drumming—a protocol later called *Health*RHYTHMS. He began with the rhythm of breathing to put people at ease by having them tune into the body. He then led the group in rhythm icebreakers, drumming the rhythms of their names, call and response, a drum circle of free expression, and guided imagery while drumming. It worked: results of blood samples showed that the new group-drumming protocol enhanced immune function significantly on a cellular level. In just one hour, the subjects transformed their biology, boosting elements of the body's natural immune system and simultaneously reducing the biochemicals that can lead to illness and disease.[8]

The study created the first evidence-based drum-circle protocol and demonstrated the advantage of participating in rhythm over just listening or "chilling out." Replicating the experiment in another part of the world, Japanese researchers tested a group of stressed-out employees, taking blood samples before and after the group-drumming protocol. Results successfully replicated Bittman's study, showing a cross-cultural truth to the health-enhancing impact of rhythm on the body.[9]

Taken together, these studies indicate a common theme. It was the active participation in drumming that boosted biology. Changing our health or enhancing our wellness requires an active role. Active drumming brings with it the health benefits of exercise, self-expression, and a sense of camaraderie and support with other drummers in the group. The study also demonstrated the accessibility of rhythm, since none of the subjects had ever played music before.

The next time flu season or allergy season approaches, it may be time to join a drum circle. Whenever we need to boost our immune system and reduce stress, we might want to consider a drum instead of a drug. The effectiveness is well documented. For more information, visit the USA Drum Circle Finder at drumcircles.net/circlelist.html.

Since Bittman's initial experiment, there have been four additional studies on group drumming, all of which were published in peer-reviewed journals. The *Health*RHYTHMS group-drumming protocol developed for Bittman's experiment has been shown to reduce employee burnout,[10] decrease anger in adolescents in corrective institutions,[11] improve mood states and participation in seniors,[12] and reduce the impact of stress in nursing students in the academic setting.[13] These studies continue to point to the functional use of rhythm across a variety of populations.

Rhythm's Work Out

The field of exercise psychology has also been examining how rhythm influences physical performance. Music obviously enhances motivation when exercising, but does it actually improve our performance when working out at the gym or going for a jog?

Costas Karageorghis, PhD, author of *Inside Sport Psychology* and head of the Music in Sport and Exercise Research Group at Brunel University, is a researcher as well as a musician who plays piano and performs in a jazz trio around London. He brought live music to mass-participation running events, such as London's half-marathon "Run to the Beat." With the success of his marathon project, Karageorghis turned into a recording artist, creating audio recordings for running that are based on scientific findings of how music can best improve our body's performance.

Karageorghis found that there is a real measurable benefit when movement is synchronized with musical tempo. He showed that when music is synchronized in rhythm to the movement rate of exercise, a 15 percent increase in treadmill endurance occurs, when compared with a control group.[14] Karageorghis also found that participant-preferred music resulted in the most significant benefits. Just imagine what you could do with 15 percent more energy in your workout!

In another study, Karageorghis compared different tempos of music at different levels of exercise intensity with regular exercisers. Results showed that a medium-to-fast tempo range of 125 to 140 beats per minute was ideal for exercise when working out in the exercise range of 40 to 90 percent maximum heart rate.[15] Tempo made a real difference. Just think of Michael Jackson's "Thriller" for medium tempo and Ritchie Valens's "La Bamba" on the faster tempo side. In most cases, for the average workout, it's best to match the tempo of the rhythm to movement.

These scientific studies give credibility to what indigenous cultures have always known: drumming is powerful medicine for the body.

The Spirit of Rhythm

Rhythm is woven into the roots of spirituality across the world. According to Navajo elders, "The drum is the Creator's favorite instrument. That's why everyone has a heartbeat."[16] Likewise, the great Nigerian drum master Babatunde Olatunji wrote the chant "I am the drum. You are the drum. We are the drum."[17]

Rhythm holds strong spiritual symbolism for shamans, who rode their drums as if they were traveling on horseback to the invisible realms of the upper and lower worlds, where they collected spirit helpers, messages, and medicine for members of the tribe facing illness. Buddhist lamas and monks play *chod* drums in ceremonies that feed demons and thus carry on ancient shamanic roots. In the words of Grateful Dead percussionist Mickey Hart, "The excitement we feel when we hear the drumbeat tells us this is the skeleton key that opens the door into the realm of Spirit."[18] Whether through trance or repeated rhythm, we enter the gate to the realm between heaven and earth, the dance hall of the spiritual world.

When I first traveled to Japan, I was amazed by the large *taiko* drums in the Buddhist temples and Shinto shrines. I learned that throughout Japanese history, as well as in the living tradition practiced today, taiko drumming is the soundtrack of ceremonial gatherings, like the church organ in European traditions. Working in Japan over the past decade, I've been invited to dance and drum in many village celebrations and ceremonies. From the Sakura Matsuri cherry blossom festivals to the August ceremony honoring ancestors in the Bön festival, all have a drumming component that uses specific rhythms to call to the spirits and nature. Japanese taiko drummers say, "The sound of the drum calls the gods to Earth to celebrate."[19]

The drum calls the tribe and holds the pulse of ceremony in many traditions. In Native American, African, Brazilian, and South American rituals, the drum represents the heartbeat of the ritual. In much of Africa, the drums anoint a sense of the sacred, whether it's in a temple, in a church, or more often, in a ceremonial space in nature. An instant temple is created by rhythm. Wherever the drum is played with intention or prayer, it creates sacred space.

Shiva's Drum

In the Hindu tradition, Shiva Nataraja, the lord of the dance, represents rhythm. This deity personifies the spiritual symbolism of the drum as a holy instrument. In one hand, Shiva holds a double-headed hourglass drum, the *damaru,* which keeps the time of the universe. In the other hand is a flame, reminding us of the creative fire and the heat of passion invoked through rhythm and dance. The beat that marks time and organizes the universe is also a call to dance.

Rhythm of the Goddess

As a woman drummer and drum-circle facilitator, I often found myself outnumbered in the male-dominated modern drum world. Then I met and studied with Layne Redmond, an award-winning percussionist whose research has tracked women's history of drumming. I also met Allessandra Belloni, who plays the Italian tambourine and continues the tradition of sacred feminine drumming in ceremonies that honor the Black Madonna. Through their books, recordings, and concerts, these women have been instrumental in awakening divine feminine healing rhythms around the world. Through them, I felt connected to a sacred and feminine root of rhythm that helped me branch out into the world as a woman and a drummer.

According to Redmond's extensive research, goddesses from centuries ago were often depicted holding drums. She points out that for thousands of years, the frame drum or tambourine was always in the hands of women doing sacred dance, drumming in processions, or even playing in front of goddesses such as Hathor, Bast, or Astarte. Further evidence of this connection comes from an ancient statue from Ur (present-day Iraq) of a woman holding her frame drum, dating back to 2000–1900 BCE. According to Redmond, "The ringing of metal jingles and the sound of the drum have always been thought to purify, announce, and proclaim the presence of the divine."[20] One of the first drummers whose name is recorded is a woman— Lipashu, the granddaughter of a Sumerian king in Mesopotamia, who drummed at the Temple of the Moon some two thousand years ago.

Although some people relish powerful forces, others perceive these forces as having a sense of danger within them. Because drumming was used in nature-based ceremonies, it was assumed by many to be a "pagan" practice (with negative connotations). The rising Roman Catholic religion actually forbade women from drumming. Yet women refused to stop drumming, particularly at the birth of a newborn baby and for funeral ceremonies.[21] The same fears of the power of rhythm led slave owners to take drums away from African slaves and led Catholic and Protestant churches to ban drumming. Today's resurgence of spiritual drumming has overcome these challenges, once again inserting the drum into its strong role in spirituality.

Parting the Seas

There is a powerful story from the Bible believed to date back to 1500 BCE and commonly referred to as the parting of the Red Sea. According to the book of Exodus, Moses was leading the Israelites to the "promised land" while being chased by the pharaoh. When they faced the impasse at the edge of the Red Sea, it looked as if they would have to turn around. But then Moses miraculously parted the sea, and they crossed, escaping their captors as the seas closed on Pharaoh's army. According to Exodus 15:20, Miriam, the prophetess and Moses's sister, took a drum in her hand, and all the women followed her with drums and dancing. The Israelites expressed their spiritual gratitude and celebration through drum medicine. Miriam played her drum, often translated as "tambourine," and all the women did likewise.

The promised land of rhythm exists within us. Through the medicine of rhythm, we leave the mind behind and return to the body of knowledge that is the keeper of the beat. A rhythm pulls us forward, overcoming seemingly impassible waters. When we arrive at the "promised land" of our own heart's rhythm, we celebrate.

Mother Earth

The drumbeat connects our hearts to Mother Earth. A chant in earth-based circles says, "From the soul of the earth comes the beating of the drum, ever more." Particularly in Native American understanding, the earth is the heartbeat. As Lakota chief Black Elk describes,

> *Thank you for the Sacred Drum,*
> *whose round form represents the entire Universe.*
> *Whose steady strong beat*
> *is the Pulse of the heart*
> *throbbing at the center of the Universe.*[22]

Body Temple

Arthur Hull, father of the drum-circle movement, often says, "The drum is like our body; a skin stretched over a shell."[23] The heartbeat in our body temple is the drum on the altar of our lives. Our bodies become the place to experience the sacred rhythms present in the holiness of life. The drumbeat carries us there.

As a drummer for an all-night women's Long Dance ceremony, I learned how rhythms affect dancers moving for a sacred intention. Gabrielle Roth, pioneering creator of Five Rhythms, created a movement practice of prayer that connects people to the body temple. She includes flowing, staccato, chaos, lyrical, and stillness rhythms. By putting the body in motion using each of these rhythms, we can "ground" the mind (and spirit) by connecting it back to the body. The body temple is the place of spiritual expression, and rhythm is the gateway.

The Medicine of Rhythm—Drum Medicine

Through drum medicine, healing happens in the convergence of science and spirit; the principle of entrainment meets the spiritual essence of the drum. The most significant thing I've witnessed in more than fifteen years of leading workshops is that the drum shows up when people are transforming. The strong presence and vibration of the drum often underlie the sense of power being reclaimed when drumming. By leading drum circles in both personal-growth retreats and in places of great tragedy and trauma, I've seen how the drum engages even the most resistant participant and releases the emotional and physical pain held in the body.

The Last Time You Danced

During my second trip to Iraq, I led a drum circle at a women's shelter. While there, despite some initial resistance, the women came to embrace drumming and ultimately were moved to get up and dance, some for the first time after a decade of being rejected by their tribes and families.

When I arrived at the shelter, I entered the living room area, where the women were sitting in a circle. They were dressed in traditional head coverings and long skirts. It was my first time seeing the scars caused by "mercy burnings"—when women are set on fire for bringing shame or dishonor to the family. For others, the scars were more hidden, including the inner wounds of abuse and loss of tribal connections.

I approached the drum circle with great sensitivity. I began by offering small shakers to the women while I played an Iraqi drum. Resistance slowly melted away as, unconsciously, feet started to tap. A few smiles began to break through. I offered the women drums, and slowly a few started to play. Everything changed in a stunning moment when the woman who had the most severe burn scars on her face, hands, and arms picked up the largest drum and played. Her statement of courage lit a fire of permission in our circle, and all the women picked up drums and joined her. Within minutes, a few women got up and started dancing, hooking arms in a traditional Kurdish line dance as they moved around the room. I couldn't believe the level of joy and the distance traveled in the transformation from sullen faces to those of smiles and laughter. The energetic dance led to singing and more dancing, until the guards requested that we quiet down.

As the rhythms slowly faded, I saw tears flowing even through the sparkles in the women's eyes. We all sat down and took a few breaths. I tried to limit the talking, but felt it was important to process the experience, so I asked them through the translator how they felt. Heads nodded, and there were more smiles. But I wanted to go deeper. I asked, "When was the last time you danced?"

One woman held up eight fingers. She hadn't danced in eight years. Another woman held up all ten fingers. Other heads nodded. I was shocked. Given that rhythm and dance were such a part of Kurdish life, I couldn't imagine the pain of being without the medicine of movement and the rhythms of the dances. Here, they were rediscovering their rhythm and empowering their spirits through the drum. As I left the shelter, all the women thanked and kissed me, sometimes three or four times, alternating cheeks on my face in what seemed to be a rhythm and dance in and of itself.

Pulled to the Pulse

The magnetic pull to the drum breaks through resistance and the common barriers that block our own healing journey. Rhythm turns off the mind and calls to the body's primary intuition. When I worked in drug and alcohol recovery centers, I repeatedly saw how the body is pulled to the pulse. Resistant patients, who sat outside the drum circle with their arms crossed over their chests, would simultaneously be tapping their feet unconsciously. Even as they would speak out loud, "I'm not doing this stupid drum thing," their feet were already engaging in the beat.

Sometimes, the mind resists what the body knows. The mind might be filled with resistance or fear, but the body knows the medicine of the drum. When I first brought *The Healing Drum Kit* into Whole Foods Market grocery stores, I did demonstrations, offering free samples of rhythm. I sat in the Whole Body section, next to the racks of vitamins, playing the healing rhythms. Shoppers walking by were immediately drawn to the beat, unconsciously tapping their hands on shopping carts or even walking to the groove. Some people would turn around and walk away, driven by their doubting mind, while others would come and experience a cathartic moment in the discovery that even they could drum. Tune into your body's wisdom, and move toward the pulse that calls you.

Good Vibrations

Drum medicine extends beyond the powerful sound of the drumbeat and into its physical vibration. Through its vibration, the drum can be used to soothe pain or activate the energy in the cells of our bodies. I once led a drumming program for patients (and their caregivers) who were facing the challenge of multiple sclerosis. Using the drum's vibration, I demonstrated how to drum over the body where it was needed. When the caregiver and partner of a man in a wheelchair drummed over his hips, he reported feeling the circulation in his body for the first time in three months. The couple took the drum home and continued the practice as he began to feel the energy move in his legs.

Taken by Trance

Drumming and rhythm hold special powers in the area of trance. The repetition of beat patterns creates a sense of the circular—spinning like a chakra, rotating like a dervish. As we drum for longer durations, life's details fade away and we fall into the place of trance, with no thought and no mind. You know you are at that place because you lose your sense of time. Hours go by, but it feels like minutes.

Rhythm has a powerful history as a tool to induce trance in ceremony, possessions, and hypnosis. The work of Allessandra Belloni has helped preserve and record the rhythms used for healing in the ancient Italian ceremonies known as the *tarantella*. In her book *Rhythm Is the Cure,* Belloni explains how the process of repetition in rhythm, combined with the dances honoring the Black Madonna, were used to create trance ceremonies through which women were healed. Holding giant frame drums with jingles like tambourines, the drummers surrounded a person who was ill. They played the ceremonial rhythms and melodies until the healing happened; sometimes this went on for days. Today this ancient practice can be accessed in our own drumming. As often happens spontaneously in drum circles, the power of group rhythm can induce a state of trance.[24]

Be in the Moment

As a tool of wellness, one of the most significant aspects of drum medicine is in the primary spiritual teaching of the drum: if you think too much, you'll screw up. This is true for any natural body movement—if you think about every step as you walk, you will trip. Drumming is the ultimate "be here now" strategy, a deactivation of the mind's wandering into the past or future. You must be in the moment; otherwise, your playing will suffer. The drumbeat calls your mind to the "now" moment, just like the metronome calls the body to walk to the beat. We entrain our minds to the beat of now, and drumming becomes an active meditation.

Coming Full Circle

Perhaps drum medicine is the reason for the fast-growing drum-circle movement worldwide, with diverse people gathering for recreation, fun, community building, and tapping into the roots of rhythm for preventive health and community building. According to *My Generation Magazine,* published by AARP, drum circles are "among America's fastest growing holistic health trends."[25] The contagious energy of the drum draws the tribe to gather, even today. In the drum circle, there is a sense of equality and inclusivity. We all need community, creativity, and energy. All are welcome, and everyone can do it. The drum circle is a collective container for self-expression.

Leading a drum circle has its own medicine. In the drum circle, the facilitator's body becomes a conductor and echoes the group's rhythm. In my work after Hurricane Katrina in St. Bernard Parish, Louisiana, my primary healing modality of the drum circle was the invitation to pass the baton. I allowed everyone to take a turn leading the drum circle. As each person stood in the center of the drumming, you could see how being empowered to lead affected his or her body. Some danced, others gave creative cues of loud or soft dynamic modulations. In the simple act of stopping the group in one concerted 4–3–2–1–STOP, individuals who had lost everything began to feel a sense of empowerment.

Similarly, in Iraq, where the drum has a history of being used in war to signal calls to troops, the group we trained led drum circles that transformed the drums of war into the drums of peace. The practice of leading and following each other, despite a history of war, became a powerful metaphor of a new paradigm of communication in Iraq.

Final Chorus

From the wisdom of the ancients to modern science, the roots of rhythm remain. Rhythm is in you: in your body, tempo changes, and the synchronicities of life. To be in rhythm is to feel the pulsing of life. This innate connection of the body and the beat is a healing force we can all tap into—for spirituality, healing, and access to the roots of rhythm that are the common pulse of humanity.

GUIDED PRACTICES FOR THE
MEDICINE OF RHYTHM
· ·

These guided practices bring the healing medicine of rhythm into your body and your life. Take a few moments to tune into your body. Where do you feel tension that needs release? Where do you need healing or energy? Are you ready to dance and create a new groove in your life?

I call these practices your RDA—recommended drumming allowance. Explore these recipes for rhythm and see what resonates for you. The first set of exercises involves conscious listening, while the second set invites you to play or dance your rhythm by expressing. Enjoy these practices of personal transformation, health, and well-being and discover the rhythm that resonates in your own body.

Guided Practices for Conscious Listening

Listening with Your Body

(All tracks from the rhythm playlist)

From the way you feel rhythm kinesthetically in bone conduction to the way a drumbeat excites your motor system, your whole body is "listening" to rhythm. Rhythm is often background in music; but through conscious listening, you can bring it into the foreground. In the rhythm playlist, I have chosen recordings that feature drum ensembles without singing or other instruments to help you feel the primacy of the beat. Although your ears may not be as used to hearing drum music, your body will recognize this primal feeling.

Start by taking a few moments to prepare yourself to receive rhythm. Shake off any stress and let your body loosen up. Breathe deeply and exhale a releasing sound. Become an open vessel for rhythm to flow into your body. Set an intention to invite the rhythm into a particular part of your body. When I work with groups, I have people say out loud, "I'm inviting the healing of rhythm into *blank part* of my body"; then I have them place their hands on that body part to direct the rhythm energy while listening. You can use the rhythm playlist (see page 50) I designed or choose your own favorite grooves.

As you listen to the music, start by sitting absolutely still. Resist the temptation to move with the beat. This way you can circumvent the automatic pathways between the body and rhythm so that deeper healing can occur. Instead of just tapping to the beat, let the rhythm reach your body. Let it surprise you. Feel which part of your body responds. It may be subtle like your belly, kneecaps, or shoulders. Let your body take in the rhythm where it needs it most. Gradually move your body with the rhythm, or simply sit still and gently pulse with the beat. Free your body to be in rhythm in your own way.

Rhythm Awareness

Play a game of hearing the rhythm around you. Notice the unique knock on the door of a colleague at the office or the rhythm in the laughter of a child. From hearing someone tapping a pen on the desk to seeing groups of people walking in rhythm, spot the rhythm everywhere. I once sat at a stoplight beyond the point when it turned green, because I was rocking out to the beat of the turning signal. Spot life's rhythmicity and join the dance.

Cultivate an awareness of the rhythmicity of life. Begin to notice moments of entrainment and synchronicity between people and within nature. By becoming aware of how often rhythms come together naturally—how often rhythm happens to you, around you, and through you—you can start to recognize the real dance of life that is going on whether in nature or between people.

A Taste of Tradition

(Tracks 2, 4, 6)

These recordings (Kakilambe, Merengue, shiko) highlight traditional rhythms played for ceremonial, ritual, and healing purposes. Kakilambe (track 2) and shiko (track 6) are African rhythms, while merengue (track 4) is an Afro-Cuban Latin groove. Made of rich, rhythmic orchestras of high and low drums, rattles, bells, tambourines, and even talking drums, these rhythms call to mind the drum lineage and the ancient calling of the drums. Experience the ancient root of rhythm in world music that is still practiced in living traditions. Can you feel how modern rhythms have evolved from these deep sources?

Drum Massage

A drum massage allows the body to listen deeply in an act of receiving the vibration of the drum. I'll describe the practices both for self-massage and for giving a drum massage to someone else. Many massage therapists and energy workers begin with a drum massage to loosen up their clients. I recommend practicing on yourself first or finding someone to take turns with. To see a video about drum massage, search for it on youtube.com/ubdrumcircles.

Choose a hoop or frame drum with a deep tone. I use the Remo Buffalo drum. The larger the drum's diameter, the lower its pitch; I use a fourteen- or sixteen-inch drum. I recommend using a soft beater and playing the drum near but not exactly at the center. This is because the center is the point where the resonance cancels itself out, creating a deadened sound. Try playing just off-center and you will hear the sweet spot where the drum really sings.

Position the drum about two inches away from the body, but not touching the body. The key is to hold the drum so the drum's underbelly (the opposite side from where you play the drumhead) faces your body. This way the vibration goes to your body. Play a simple pulse at a comfortable tempo. In a self-massage, feel the energy and vibration against your body—the sonic ultrasound. You can concentrate on one area or do a total body clearing with the drum by holding it up over your head and then drumming down the front side of your body.

When giving a drum massage to another person, hold the drum so it vibrates toward them. Start above the person's head and work your way down the front; then repeat on the back, from head to toe. Ask where the person needs more energy, and drum a little longer where it's needed.

I've created a group practice in which everyone faces left in a circle and gives a drum massage to the back of the person in front, while simultaneously receiving the massage from the person behind. I've also had one person stand in the center encircled by drummers to create a very powerful mass drum massage. Get creative and learn to let your body receive the drum medicine.

Guided Practices for Expressing

Heartbeat

Now it's time to get out a drum or other percussion instrument and be the beat. Drumming grounds us in our bodies, tuning us into the heartbeat that is the inner drum. When you need to slow down, take time to simply play a heartbeat pulse on your drum. This simple beat is played for hours in Native American ceremonies. It is the pulse of the community and the anchor of chanting. It is what entrains the community to the heartbeat of the earth.

Tune into your heart, the center of love and life within you. Start by blessing your drum by sweeping your open hand over the drumhead in a whispered statement of gratitude and recognition of the drum's ancient path. Set your intention to be centered, grounded, and rooted in rhythm. Feel the deep heartbeat of your soul.

When you're ready, place your hand on your drum. Begin to play the pulse in your own way. It may be the beat that sounds like "lub-dub, lub-dub" or an ongoing pulse. Gradually let the beat grow and change and become more an expression of you.

Be the Beat—Become the Drum

(Tracks 10 and 11)

Join in with these play-along recordings from UpBeat Drum Circles ("Reviving Rhythms" in duple meter, "Beauty Groove" in triple meter), which have been specifically designed to help you entrain with a strong, pulsing bass drum and a bell or rattle. The contrast of high and low percussion sounds will help you fall into the groove. It takes about four minutes to deeply entrain, which is probably the time it takes to deactivate the mind and move into the body.

I often recommend using headphones or another good sound source with play-along tracks, so that your drumming doesn't overpower the music. Begin by listening to the music. Feel it in your body. Move your body without drumming. This prepares you for success as you begin to join the beat. Join the rhythm by playing a pulse at first, and gradually get out of your way enough so you are creating your own beat.

The key is this: Don't think! This is harder than it sounds. In my groups, people often comment that the minute they noticed their rhythm sounded good, just that instant of thought made them lose the beat.

This is a powerful practice for being in the moment and trusting your rhythm to come through. It's the creativity that makes a difference in empowering your body.

To extend this practice into the world, join a drum circle. There are many digital search tools to help you find a drum circle in your area—for example, drumcircle.net or remo.com/health can both help you find your way.

Mojo Moving

(All tracks)

Creative movement is the jazz of dance, and rhythm is your partner. Get out of your head and get into your body by free-dancing to the rhythms in the rhythm playlist. This type of movement is not rehearsed, and it's not about following steps. The recordings in the rhythm playlist go beyond four minutes, allowing you to fall into the groove and cross the threshold of self-doubt. Be patient with your experience, and it will unfold naturally. You can use this practice when you get home from work, when you rise in the morning, or whenever you need a break from too much thinking. As you repeat this practice, you'll notice that the same song drives a different dance each time. Dance to the beat of your own drum and get your mojo moving.

Drum Prayer

If you want to send energy to someone or someplace in the world, the drum can be your prayer partner. For centuries, prayer has been a primary use of drums in ceremony and personal spiritual practice, calling to the gods of heaven or to the four directions in nature. Indigenous cultures have known for centuries how to shape their prayers into the vibration of beauty produced within song and rhythm.

Take a moment to start by setting your intention. Center your prayer in the inner drum of your heart. Hold a moment of silence to focus your intention more deeply. What is the rhythm of the person you are praying for? What rhythm is needed: grounding and focus, or passion and creativity?

When you're ready, play a beat that represents your intention. Do not drum word phrases; rather, drum the feeling tone of the energy of your prayer. When you are finished, gradually soften your playing, falling back into silence. In the silence that follows the final beat, visualize the prayer going where it's needed, reaching the person, place, or your own heart.

ANNOTATED PLAYLIST FOR RHYTHM

To stream this music, visit SoundsTrue.com/MusicMedicine.

1. "Mountain Mist," Glen Velez, *Rhythms of Awakening*
Awaken the cells of your body to the beat of master drummer Glen Velez
playing the Remo *bodhrán,* an Irish frame drum, accompanied by shakers,
bones, and harmonica.

2. "Kakilambe in 6," KDZ (The Drummers at Kripalu, live), *Nataraja* (compiled by Shiva Rea)
Kakilambe is a West African dance rhythm. This recording embodies the feminine that causes your hips to sway in the triple meter of 6/8. This groove starts
at 108 beats per minute and gradually rises, building the energy.

3. "The Whirler," Layne Redmond, *Invoking the Muse*
Fall into trance with this invocation to the muse of dance. Ancient Middle
Eastern drums, tambourines, and triangles are played over the sound of a
bull-roarer, which is swung in a circular motion to generate a tone. Let
your body listen to the polyrhythm of three-beat triple and four-beat duple
pulses circulating together.

4. "Arroz Con Merengue," Pepe Danza, *Drum Prayers*
The Afro-Cuban dance rhythm of merengue meets the saxophone and a
choir of singers, as Joseph "Pepe" Danza plays congas, bongo, and *cajon.* Hear
the subtle rhythm of a triangle, the feeling of pause and pulse when the
drum breaks happen, and the excitement of interchange between saxophone
rhythms and drums. Enjoy this fantastic improvisational driving rhythm that
harkens to the pulse of Latin rhythm.

5. "Citric Motion," Glen Velez, *Rhythms of Awakening*
In a complex rhythm that moves between six- and five-beat rhythms, this
rich polyrhythm has a sacred combination of tambourine jingles, a frame
drum (*tar*), and a *bansuri* Indian flute played by Steve Gorn. A simple chant at
the end invites the voice into the body groove.

6. "Shiko," Geoff Johns, *Bakongo!*
Recorded by Geoff Johns's ensemble, this Nigerian rhythm is made to
dance, to pulse your body into rhythm. You can hear the sound of a talking
drum literally speaking in the pitches of a small, double-headed drum that is
played by squeezing it under the armpit to tense and loosen the outer strings.
At a tempo of 130 beats per minute, this driving African rhythm features an
ensemble of drums and bells. It's pure rhythm!

7. "Naomba Ukuwe Mazuri," Shaman's Dream, *African Dream*
Inspired by a trip to Kenya and Tanzania, this recording is in the 6/8 rhythm,
leading you to sway your hips. Balophones, which are xylophones with
gourd resonators, join rattles, drums, and the sounds of animals and nature.

8. "The Proclaimer," Layne Redmond, *Invoking the Muse*
Shimmering with the jingles of three drums—tambourine, the Remo Tar-Rine,
and the Brazilian *pandeiro*—Layne Redmond brings us into rhythm with an
invocation proclaiming the glory of the muse and the groove of the body. Feel
this interesting pulse that follows the 3–3–2 pattern.

9. "Secret Messenger," Glen Velez, *Breathing Rhythms*
Tune into the sounds of Irish bodhrán, rattles, cello, pan flutes, and the
spoken syllables "Na Ka Ta Ri Ki Ta Ta Ka." Percussionist Glen Velez is
joined by cellist Eugene Friesen and pan flutist Damian Dragichi. Tune into
the secret messenger of rhythm that speaks to your body.

10. "Reviving Rhythms," Christine Stevens, *The Healing Drum Kit*
Join in the beat with this medium-tempo play-along track for your personal
rhythmical expression. The recording is mixed specifically for you to join
the rhythm with your *own* thing or to dance with your *mojo* motion.

11. "Beauty Groove," Christine Stevens, *Drumming Up Diva—
Women's Empowerment Drumming*
This play-along recording features a triple meter or 6/8 groove to move your
hips as you dance to the music, or you can play along with your own drum
or favorite percussion instrument. Featuring a sweet, improvised melody on a
flute, this track was recorded with a powerful team of women drummers!

4

Melody: Medicine for the Heart

When you feel down and out
Sing a song, it'll make your day
Here's a time to shout
Sing a song, it'll make a way.

—EARTH, WIND, AND FIRE, "SING A SONG"

There is a reason that even in places of war, suffering, and loss, songs keep singing. Melodies that live in our hearts can never be taken away. They serve our need for expression, heart connection, and healing. Melody speaks the language of the heart.

When I returned from working in St. Bernard Parish after Hurricane Katrina in New Orleans, I experienced a kind of depression known as compassion fatigue, which is common in crisis workers. Witnessing such devastation and depression had deeply touched me. I couldn't concentrate, I had low energy, and I felt a weight on my heart that I couldn't shake. I experienced an overwhelming sense that as much as I tried to help, so much more was needed.

About a week later, a simple phrase started to sing in my mind: "Music can't be washed away." It was inspired by a man I had met while singing to people in the long, slow line at the Federal Emergency Management Agency (FEMA) office. He was a musician who had lost three guitars in the hurricane, but he rolled up his sleeve and pointed to a tattoo of a guitar on his upper arm and said, "This is the only guitar that Katrina couldn't wash away." I nodded, pointed to his heart, and said, "And this is the real instrument behind the music. Katrina could not take it away either."

I thought about how nothing can take away the music within us. No war, tragedy, conflict, or oppression. I sat at the piano and started singing. The words *music can't be washed away* eventually became a song. Hours went by. With each line, I felt the weight released from my heart, and I felt my mood improve. I was singing my way through the healing moments of my time working with the people who had lost everything, yet who still had hope. It worked; my symptoms went away. The song became the healing medicine I needed—a homeopathic remedy of the song medicine within my own heart.

I experienced compassion fatigue again, years later, after my second trip to northern Iraq in 2008. That year, we had toured the Kurdish Genocide Museum, which was housed in one of Saddam Hussein's former torture centers. The experience was particularly heartfelt because our translator, Lydia, had actually fled during the exile into the mountains in 1992, running from the torture and fearing for her life. When I returned home from Iraq, I immediately recognized the symptoms of compassion fatigue and started singing. I sang about the pain, confusion, and injustice, and slowly I began to feel better. "A Beat for Peace" was the song and melody I wrote for my own healing. Through melody, I released the burden around my heart and set my heart free again to hope, love, and gratitude. A video of this song, recorded live in Iraq, can be found by searching for it at youtube.com/ubdrumcircles.

Heartstrings

Notes open the gateways of our hearts. We are moved by the melody that touches, soothes, awakens, releases, or inspires our heart centers. We know when a melody reaches our heartstrings because tears come and emotions that sometimes surprise us burst forth. It's not a cognitive process; it's about feeling.

Our expressions show the connection between melody and the heart. When music is memorized, we say we know it by heart. When we belt out a tune, we say we're singing our hearts out. We listen to our heart song, and hearing our favorite song plays on our heartstrings. The term *heartstring* actually comes from the *chordae tendineae,* which are the tendons that open and close the heart valves.

When we speak, there is a melody in language arts; this melody is the spoken song that sings of our emotions. Linguists call this melody of our language *prosody*—the high and low pitches, the rising and falling melodic contour that underscores our words. The melody of language communicates the emotions of our hearts. It's the song in the notes of language that sing the feelings behind our words. In human development, melody predates language; we sing before we speak. Perhaps instead of the African saying "If you can talk, you can sing," the reverse may be truer: "If you can sing, you can talk."

Melody is a powerful healing force that allows us to move more deeply into a place of love that is a genesis of healing. Heart-centeredness is a metaphor of living from compassion and passion, no longer cut off from the juice that drives music's serenading force of love. You might say that melody is a form of open-heart surgery. As Sufi master Hazrat Inayat Khan said, "If one can focus one's heart on music, it is just like warming something that was frozen. The heart returns to its natural condition."[1]

Broken Hearts

Whether we have a broken heart from loss or relationship or we have a physical heart problem, both emotional and physical heart centers are often in need of healing. Sometimes a closed heart needs to be broken open in cathartic moments so that feelings that have burdened our hearts are finally released.

The Beatles sang that money can't buy you love, but can it buy you happiness? It turns out that the happiest countries in the world are not necessarily the wealthiest ones. According to psychologist Adrian White of the University of Leicester in the United Kingdom, who created the World Map of Happiness, the United States ranks twenty-third in happiness, which is far behind Denmark (first), Switzerland (second), the Bahamas (fifth), or Canada (tenth).[2] It makes me wonder whether the pursuit of wealth that seems to define Western culture has replaced the pursuit of happiness, love, and joy, which are the emotions that cause our hearts to sing.

Modern life poses challenges to creating and maintaining relationships that bring love into our hearts. In America, only thirty-eight percent of married people surveyed in 1996 rated their marriage as happy.[3] Half of American marriages end in divorce, but that doesn't stop us from trying.

Second and third marriages show even higher rates of divorce—sixty-seven percent for second and seventy-four percent for third marriages.[4]

Our hearts are currently under great strain from a rise in both stress and weight gain. An estimated 76.4 million adults in the United States have stress-related hypertension; of those, 71 percent are using antihypertensive medication.[5] These conditions are rising at alarming rates, even in people of early age. In the United States, 34 percent of individuals aged twenty or younger already have hypertension. Heart disease is on the rise. Approximately every twenty-five seconds, an American will have a coronary incident, and approximately every minute, someone will die from one. Heart disease is one of the leading causes of death worldwide, and accounts for 25 percent of all deaths in the United States annually, according to the Centers for Disease Control and Prevention.

Take a moment to consider your own heart, both physically and energetically. Where in your heart do you need healing? How often are you in touch with joy, love, happiness, and the notes that make your heart sing? How often do you repress the emotions of your heart? How often do you really listen to your heart?

The Art of Melody

We all have a unique melody—our individual sound print, the song of who we are, the melodic force that brings our authentic voice to the symphony of life. After we are incubated in rhythm, we are born in melody, sounding our cry of life into the world. The voice is connected to the throat chakra, which represents communication. The word *voice* shares the same Latin root (*vocalis*) as the word *vocation*. When we feel that our voice is heard and empowered in our life's work, a sense of authentic presence in the larger workforce of the world is created. It could be said that finding your voice is reflected in living the song of your purpose.

Melody is defined as a series of notes that create a sweet arrangement of sound. It's the sweetness and the uniqueness that create the "hook" in a song and the pull on our heartstrings. Composers hear it, cantors express prayers through it, and children learn their ABCs with it. Melody creates jazz, jingles that sell products, classical themes and variations, chants and hymns of faith, and rock tunes.

Melodies are built from scales, shaped by contour, composed by heart, and sung to life by vocalists and instruments. Musical scales underlie melodies like the scaffolding of buildings. Scales create different tonalities that touch our emotions. Scales may be major, which sound bright or happy, or minor, which can sound sad, pensive, or mournful. They may be eight notes, like "do, re, mi, fa, so, la, ti, do" taught in *The Sound of Music* song. Five-note pentatonic scales comprise five notes that are the black keys on the piano. You recognize pentatonic scale–based melodies in gospel music, African slave songs, Native American flute scales, and Asian-sounding compositions. The beauty of pentatonic scales is that their open, expansive tonality allows no wrong notes. I call it the "freedom scale," because it allows improvisation without the fear of making a bad sound.

Scales speak the sonic identity of different world cultures—whether they are Japanese, Balinese, Iraqi microtonal scales, or the Kurdish scale I became familiar with in Iraq. In the Middle East, melodies come from microtonal scales with quarter-tones, which are very difficult to hear with Western ears. In India, ragas are like scales; they are series of notes that match the spirit and energy of a purpose, time of day, or specific emotion. There is a raga for love, devotion, kindness, honoring a great teacher, and so on. For example, the raga *Hansa-bwani*, meaning "two swans," is a heart raga of five notes associated with love and the heart center.

Wordless Song

Melody is a language of the heart that can communicate emotions that words alone cannot say. If you've ever been touched by a wordless melody in jazz or classical compositions, without knowing what it meant, you've felt the medicine of melody. Without language, melody births classical themes and variations, jazz tunes, and world music compositions. The sound of a flute melody or cello reaches our hearts more easily than words because there is less thought involved. *(Listen to tracks 1, 3, and 10 in the melody playlist.)*

A form of melody that's in between word and wordlessness is scatting. Jazz vocalists use nonsense syllables to improvise in the instrument of the voice. Scat singing is made famous by singers whose hearts can speak in melody.

Four Meanings of Melody

Melodies create access to the four healing properties of song. Songs reflect deep heart emotions and create touchstones to the most important moments of our lives.

1. *Opening.* A closed heart can feel restricted, tight, and burdened. Holding onto resentment and pain, our hearts become discouraged, depressed, and even bitter. The medicine of melody allows a release of the burdens that we hold in our hearts. Heaviness is transformed to lightness. We may not even know what caused our heart pain or what we were holding onto, but we can feel when it's released. Sometimes a song says exactly how we feel, and we have an immediate sense of relief upon hearing it sung. Even wordless melodies can tell a heart's story and mirror the emotions that our heart is longing to tell.

2. *Empowering.* Before the team goes on the field or warriors go into battle, they gather and chant. Melody empowers our energy, our truth, and our authentic voice. From the beauty and uniqueness that each of us is here to express to the common song that bonds groups, melody strengthens us. No one can ever take a song away from you.

In some tribal villages in Africa, a pregnant mother goes to see the shaman, who listens to the song of the baby's soul in the mother's womb. Once the baby is born, the whole village gathers to sing the melody that has been taught by the shaman to the mother. Imagine being born into your heart song.

Chanting someone's name in a healing way empowers that person's spirit. In my workshops, I often invite one person into the center of the circle; then I have everyone chant that person's name. People's names create an opportunity to sing their hearts back to them and surround them in song.

3. *Remembering.* From learning information to recalling rich experiences, melody harnesses the power of memory. Songs are well-documented mnemonic tools helping us learn things "by heart." It's funny how we often can't remember our ABCs without singing them. From mathematical formulas, alphabets, and state capitals to important rules to live by in the oral traditions of tribal cultures, melody is a carrier wave of remembrance. Seniors come alive when they hear the songs they fell in love to. Patients with Alzheimer's disease remember lyrics to favorite hymns, despite severe memory loss. Hearing a certain song on the radio can take you back to that precious moment in your life. Melodies are time-travel machines, helping our hearts become young again in song.

Because melody is such a strong medicine for remembering, a song can get stuck in our minds. Researchers call this the "earworm" effect. Studies show that this phenomenon is surprisingly common: 90 percent of people experience an earworm at least every week.[6] Once it's in you, a song can be difficult to dislodge. On the upside, songs help us pass tests, learn information, and remember facts and figures. On the downside, songs in advertising jingles call us to buy things. You have to decide whether you want to hear the melody that makes your heart sing or the one that makes you want to shop.

4. *Soothing.* A peaceful melody played softly and slowly creates comfort and calm for a restless heart. The right song pulls our heart's attention away from fear or from feeling unsettled and helps us return to peace and calm. The melodies of lullabies are one of the most universal song forms practiced worldwide. In fact, lullabies from all over the world have a common musical structure, regardless of language or culture. Their melodies are repetitive, have a slow tempo, and have a limited pitch range. What soothes us in music is universal to humanity.

The Shape of Your Heart

Remember the old sing-along technique of "follow the bouncing ball"? Karaoke machines use this method to guide us through the melodies of songs, making the auditory melody a visual picture. It's the rise and fall in the movement from note to note that forms melodic contour and shapes our emotions. Like a pumping heart, melodies expand and contract, creating the breadth and the breath of melody, the life force of song that reaches our hearts. Note-to-note movement changes from baby steps in tight intervals to giant leaps in wide intervals. Life is lived in moments of contrast. The highs and lows of notes mirror the rise and fall of the heart's emotions. The ups and downs move us.

Even as melody carries our heart in the tune's own unique adventure, there is a longing to return to where we began. In melody, the home note is called the root or tonic. Repetition creates predictability, but fluctuation creates surprise; it's the yin and yang of song that mirrors life's emotions. At the end of any journey, we feel moved by coming back home—settled and solid, grounded and complete.

The Principle of Melody—Song Alchemy

Songs ignite a creative fire that can alchemize feelings and literally "take a sad song and make it better." Songs born of struggle often transform hearts from fear and despair to hope and inspiration. The songs of African slaves gave hope to aching hearts longing for freedom. Spiritual songs, like "Wade in the Water" and "Freedom Is Coming," were not sung for entertainment, but for emotional and spiritual survival, holding tight to a sonic chord of hope that could not be taken away by any form of capture.

One of the greatest stories of the alchemy of song is the origin of "Amazing Grace." John Newton was the captain of a ship transporting slaves from Africa to the New World. One evening, a storm grew violent at sea, and Newton feared he would lose his life. That dark storm became a catalyst for a prayer that led him to renounce his life and change his ways. Newton survived and later became a preacher and activist for the abolition of slavery. He went from slave trader to minister, and with his heart born anew in the grace of redemption, he began writing songs. In 1772, John Newton wrote lyrics to a melody he most likely learned from slaves singing in pentatonic scales, which later became the hymn "Amazing Grace." It tells the story of how he received his sight, his vision, and most importantly his authentic voice. He literally changed his tune.

Chains around our hearts can enslave our emotions and cause us to shut down. Shame, guilt, blame, and regret can all capture us in an emotional prison of our own creation. Our hearts may become wrapped in fear or be unable to let go and trust again. As a music therapist, I witnessed the power of individuals breaking free of their own inner heart prison. Using blues melodies rewritten by clients is a wonderfully effective therapy for overcoming abuse, alcoholism, or depression.

Songs that hold meaning to our hearts bring forth tears in the same way that rhythm commands the body to move. In song, we move through difficult times in our lives. In song alchemy, the wounded heart can be transformed to a heart of gold, the way metal is transformed to gold in alchemy. Even the act of singing transforms breath to song.

The Shadow Side of Melody

The power of melody can go both ways. Melody can also misguide us, be used for propaganda, and, in some extreme cases, cause us to lose our way and forget our own tune. In Greek mythology, the shadow of song is represented in the Sirens' song. Often identified as the muses of the underworld, the Sirens play the harp and flute and sing in a trio of such beautiful music that sailors are seduced by song and captured on the island, never to be seen again.

How do we resist or conquer the shadow side of melody? Greek mythology gives two examples. Odysseus put wax in the ears of his crew, but he left his ears open to hear the Sirens' song. He had himself bound to the mast, with strict instructions not to let him go. As they passed the Sirens' island and the song wafted into Odysseus's ears, he begged to be released as expected, but the crew refused, tying him even tighter. Odysseus demonstrated a powerful practice: we can listen to a seductive melody, but only if we resolve to remain where we are and not leave our post, literally, to chase the Sirens' song.

In another myth, Orpheus plays his own music so beautifully that the ship's crew cannot hear the song of the Sirens. His music overpowers the Sirens' alluring sound. Sometimes, we need to strengthen our own song to counteract the powerful pull of the Sirens' song.

Being true to our inner melody holds us steady in our center. The most important song is the one that leads us forward to ourselves in the ultimate path of true power and discovery of our own heart song. Be aware of the impact of song. When you are stuck in a dark place, notice whether adopting a new song can help change your tune.

The Science of Melody

Our instinctive connection to melody is part of its medicine in our lives. Child-development researchers have discovered remarkable evidence of our earliest years of development being filled with an innate capacity for melody and song. Even if you're tone-deaf or feel you "can't carry a tune in a bucket," scientifically we are all wired for song.

Our Innate Sense of Song

Our ears are the first sensory organs to develop at four months into gestation. For five months in utero, we are listening in the concert hall of the womb, surrounded by amniotic fluid that serves as an amplifier, doubling the volume. Given this degree of amplification, you may wonder how much sound we absorb. Is there music we hear in utero that we can recognize even after birth?

A study by Peter G. Hepper at Queens University in Belfast, Ireland, looked at the degree to which music heard in utero could be recognized and remembered.[7] Hepper used the theme songs of popular television shows watched by pregnant mothers months before the birth to see how much newborn babies could recognize the tunes. Sure enough, just two to four days after birth, newborn babies recognized the theme songs. They became calm, showed a decrease in heart rate and movement, and became more alert, compared to a lack of response to unfamiliar theme songs.

Two conclusions can be drawn from this study. First, it seems that early on, our sense of song is already highly attuned. We remember and recognize melody early in our lives. Second, if you're pregnant, be aware of the songs and sounds in your environment after five months' gestation. Not only are you eating for two, but you are listening for two as well.

In a follow-up study, Hepper found that as they age, babies develop even finer-tuned song recognition. In an experiment, six-month-olds to one-year-olds recognized changes in notes, order of notes, and rhythms of notes between familiar and unfamiliar melodies. In a similar study, researchers had parents play a CD of two folk melodies in major and minor keys for three minutes a day over a period of seven straight days. Amazingly, the infants could already differentiate the folk melodies they heard from unfamiliar ones.[8] Before age one, we are fast learners and have a highly attuned sense of song.

To see just how well babies could recognize songs, in both studies the researchers made it more challenging by playing the familiar melodies in different keys—what musicians call *transposition,* putting the same melodic contour in a higher or lower position. Remarkably, the infants were not fooled and still recognized the familiar melodies. This finding led researchers to believe that it's the contour of the melody more than the individual notes that help us recognize melodies. However, the voice of the melody does matter. The research also found that the actual sound of the instrument producing the melody needed to be consistent for recognition. This makes sense, given that our highly attuned ears help us recognize the sonic quality of the voices of significant people in our lives.

Dr. Sandra Trehub at the Infant and Child Studies Center at Toronto University made an interesting discovery: even before the age of one, we can name that tune in six notes. She tested eleven-month-old infants by playing a six-note melody for twenty minutes. She wondered whether the infants could distinguish the tunes from unfamiliar melodies without repeated exposure. Indeed, after just twenty minutes of listening, the infants were able to recognize the melodies, even when those songs were transposed to higher or lower keys.[9]

Our Songwriting Instinct

Not only do we recognize melodies with great accuracy, we are all innately songwriters. If you've ever doubted that you were musical or creative, reading this research will give you the confidence that there is a song in your heart that wants to be expressed.

Peter Ostwald, MD, of the University of California San Francisco Medical Center, studied children's natural musicality, which comes without training, teaching, or modeling. He found that children as early as six months old demonstrate spontaneous singing of their own original melodies, without songwriting having been modeled or taught by their parents.[10]

Think about it. Your parents probably didn't walk around making up songs. That usually only happens at the opera or on the television show *Glee*. Songwriting seems to be an innate and instinctive part of human development. By age two to three, as their vocabulary grows, children demonstrate even greater ability to make up their own songs, forming choruses and compositions to express their emotions and joyful experiences in life. If you're lucky, you've caught a child making up a song about anything from riding the bus to playing around a tree. It's quite extraordinary and full of creative spirit. Perhaps this innate call to create song is what birthed the "play songs" that are the soundtrack of playgrounds. When we are most full of joy, the heart wants to sing. Playfulness generates creativity, an important principle to remember as adults.

To tie the notes of these research studies together, we see strong evidence that we are all naturally attuned to song. As infants, we recognize melodies, learn melodies, and create our own melodies. But if songwriting is so innate, what stops us from composing and singing our heart songs as adults? How do we lose touch with the brave singing spirit that is so innate within us all? How can we access our inner two-year-old songwriter and our natural drive for fearless self-expression?

Singing Your Heart Out

Even though we may not be professional singers, we can all use melody to strengthen our physical hearts through the breath that becomes song, what

I call *prana-melodica*. Breath is important to our hearts. As adults, we become busy and often hurry through our day, running the risk of literally getting out of breath. Our blood becomes less oxygenated. Stress can cause shallow breathing, which decreases lung capacity, which can lead to greater risk of heart disease. In a longitudinal population study, lung capacity was found to be a significant predictor of heart problems, stroke, respiratory disease, cancer, and other causes of death—second only to cholesterol levels. The study excluded individuals who smoked or were obese, showing that even healthy "normal" people need to pay attention to breathing.[11]

A New Zealand study looked at whether changes in lung capacity at a young age could predict future heart problems. The study found that decreased lung capacity correlated with increased heart disease. It also discovered that this correlation takes place at a young adult age, much earlier than previously thought. The connection between how we breathe and our heart health seems clear, and singing can be a pathway to better breathing.[12]

When we make music, the health benefits are even greater than when we listen. When we sing, we engage our physical bodies, improving lung capacity and getting an aerobic workout that benefits our heart. A study by Gunter Kreutz at Oldenburg University in Germany used saliva samples and subjective surveys of emotional states to compare singing choral music with listening to it. He found significant improvement in immune system markers, including immunoglobulin A and cortisol, as well as affective improvement only in the singing condition.[13]

Singing is a healthy workout that tones the chest-wall muscles and improves respiration, in a manner similar to swimming, rowing, and even yoga. Kathleen McCormick, a nurse and researcher at the National Institute on Aging's Gerontology Research Center, studied heart and lung function in twenty opera singers and compared them with a control group of nonsingers.[14] Although lung capacity generally declines with age, she found that the opera singers had stronger chest-wall muscles and greater lung capacity. This result was surprising, given that many of the singers did not exercise and some even smoked. The vocalists' hearts pumped blood more efficiently, and their heart rates were lower.

In a study using respiratory kinematics (a technique that studies the motions of the chest wall) and respiratory electromyographic (EMG) analysis of lung measurements, college students who were enrolled in singing lessons over three semesters demonstrated improved lung-volume expansion, rib cage expansion, and abdominal capacity. There was even greater health improvement as the students progressively increased their singing volume and pitch range—the more intense the volume and range of song, the more exercise these interior muscles get.[15] When your heart is ready to sing, sing loud!

In summary, studies show how the medicine of melody is innate within us all from our first days of life. The song inside you and the breath that supports its expression strengthen your heart. From the emotional connection of the baby's cooing to the mother's matched sounds, melody brings our hearts together. Not only is melody a medicine of communication between mother and child, melody can also guide and open our hearts toward the spiritual.

The Spirit of Melody

The innate human drive to create melody is ancient and unwavering. Our hearts have driven us to chant and pray in melodies for thousands of years, using the oldest instrument: the human voice. Historically, tribal cultures used song and chant as tools for spiritual connection in shamanic traditions. Although few written records remain, African chants passed down orally have taught spiritual wisdom and put affirmations of healing into song. A Nigerian chant taught by Babatunde Olatunji says *"ara mi le,"* which means, "I am well, my body is well."

Chanting and singing are universal entry points into the spiritual realms. Rabbi Pinchas of Koretz, an eighteenth-century scholar of the Zohar (a mystical interpretation of the Jewish Talmud), wrote, "There is a temple in heaven that is only opened through song."[16]

The power of song for spiritual connection is also embodied in the Lakota creation story of "First Born," as written by Ruth Beebe Hill in her novel *Hanta Yo.* Notice the importance of rhythm and song, the two aspects of music's medicine that we have been exploring thus far. We awaken both the beat and the song, both the rhythm and the melody, as a sound pathway to the power of the Spirit.

First Born, the Grandfathers told, had emerged from quivering mud to the rhythm of his own heart, and so man had known the true rhythm from the beginning. Soon afterwards, man had learned to use this rhythm for making songs. And then certain ones had discovered the true power in song; the power for making spiritual contact.[17]

Morning Song

The morning song holds a universal place in spiritual traditions as the practice of the call to prayer or of greeting the day. Navajo call the deity of the morning Dawn Woman. Tibetans chant at sunrise to Ozen Chagma, the Goddess of the Spreading Dawn Rays. The Cherokee face east and sing "The Morning Song" over the heartbeat rhythm on the drum. The translation of the lyrics *"We n' de ya ho, He ya ho, He ya ho, Ya ya ya"* means "I am of the Great Spirit." Dawn is also the time of the first call to prayer that is chanted in mosques throughout the Islamic world. When I was in Iraq and in the Muslim lands of the Far East, the call to prayer chanting the Quran permeated the air at dawn, wafting into empty streets and slumbering homes, broadcast through loudspeakers from the minarets. What a beautiful wake-up call to the heart.

How do you start the day? Can you bring a morning song into your personal spiritual practice as an expression of gratitude, a new beginning, and a connection to the heart?

Ceremony in Song

Songs and chants amplify our intentions, beautify prayers, and are part of ancient traditions still practiced today. Through spending time with Lakota teachers, I continue to learn songs that speak to the heart of all life. These songs communicate with the natural world in the call to the four directions and the call to the Creator. Songs thank the elements of wind, water, stones, and the earth. In Lakota culture, prayer songs hold an important purpose in ceremony. Welcoming songs ring out as the ceremony begins, while gratitude songs are sung at the closing. Songs set the ceremony's tone and speak its heartfelt intention. Singers serve the community by becoming song keepers and, in this way, lead the medicine chants that unite us. When we depart from the ceremony, the songs travel with us, creating a blanket of comfort in the transition from ceremony to real-world living. Our songs are the sap of the spiritual community we have built, and they are preserved in the heart. Whenever I sing or hear these songs, the feeling tone of that empowering experience is reawakened in my heart.

Enchanted

Song and chant are a universal part of spiritual traditions. According to Benedictine monk Brother David Steindl-Rast, "Chanting is an integral part of all the world's religious traditions—Buddhist, Jewish, Hindu, Islamic, and others. At a certain pitch of religious experience, the heart just wants to sing; it breaks into song."[18]

The word *enchant* and the word *chant* share the root word *contare*, which means "to sing." The melodies of chants create a repetition of beauty, a recapitulation of the sacred that fills the deep places in the heart's longing for spiritual union. It's no wonder that most religious services begin with chanting or congregational singing. Melody in the form of spiritual chanting reverberates with gratitude, joy, and prayer, drawing us into the heart and our connection with the Divine.

Kirtan, a form of ecstatic call-and-response chanting, is a practice of devotion from the bhakti yoga tradition of eastern India. Chants repeat the names of the Hindu deities. Paramahansa Yogananda, founder of the Self-Realization Fellowship, was a prolific composer of devotional chants. He wrote, "Listen, listen, listen to my heart song. I will never forget Thee. I will never forsake Thee."[19] The spirit of melody brings us back to the heart song—the place of love, devotion, and spiritual practice of the heart. Whether starting the day with a morning song, chanting in a group, or singing prayer songs to start a religious service, through the spirit of melody, we evoke our heart center, bypass the mind, and attune ourselves to a vibration of the divine. *(Listen to tracks 6, 7, and 8 in the melody playlist to hear kirtan recordings.)*

Love's Song

The ancient art of serenading a lover is an archetypal ritual of courtship. Even in our time of computers, texting, speed-dating, and online dating, there is an ancient tradition of singing to capture the heart of a loved one—a melodic drive that cannot be extinguished by digital methods. People still dedicate songs to those they love, or they email song files to communicate their love.

This same desire applies to the melodies of devotion to the Divine. The practice of singing a rich melody of love to enchant a partner's heart is no different from the act of courting God. One of the greatest uses of melody is in the hymns and chants that call from our hearts to the Divine, wooing the presence of love and beauty.

Krishna's Flute

Instruments can also sing the heart awake. The flute can open the hearts of both the player and the listener. I often play the Native American flute in the hospital rooms of cancer patients, witnessing the sense of heart awakening, soothing, peacefulness, and relief from pain it brings.

Flutes are one of the oldest instruments unearthed in archaeological digs. An ancient five-hole flute carved out of bird bone, found in the Hohle Fels cave in southwest Germany, dates back some thirty-five thousand years to the Stone Age.[20] Amazingly, the notes of the flute had similar intervals to those of modern-day instruments.

Iconic spiritual flutists from the traditions of different world religions represent the divine melody-playing archetype. In India, Hindu deity Krishna played his golden flute, attracting cowherd women, called *gopis,* who fell in love with him and, dancing in enchantment, left their work and followed him. The mythological Kokopelli, a Native American fertility symbol, is said to have played his flute to capture the hearts of women. Both icons carry a similar message—sweet, heartfelt flute melodies create a connection with the Divine and a magnetic call to the spiritual heart. Perhaps the greatest spiritual love may be best spoken through song.

The Native American flute is often called the love flute because of the story of its creation. It is said that a young man longing for a beautiful girl was rejected by her and went off into the woods, filled with sorrow. He walked for so long that he eventually grew tired and fell asleep under a large cedar tree. In his dream, he heard a sweet, contagious melody. He awoke, humming its tune, only to discover that the notes he heard were mysteriously coming from the tree. While he was sleeping, a woodpecker, out of compassion for the young boy, had made holes in a tree branch and asked the wind to blow and play the notes. The young man learned to carve the flute and play the melody and then returned to the village to play his song to the young girl. Upon hearing the melody, she immediately fell in love with him and accepted his admiration.

The Medicine of Melody—Song Medicine

The power in the medicine of melody is taking the innate sense of song and songwriting and applying it to healing, self-care, and personal growth. As a music therapist working in the area of addiction, I used songwriting with clients, many of whom associated music with their drug or alcohol experiences. Songwriting allowed them to literally change their tune.

One of the strongest moments of song medicine happened while I was working with Arthur, an agitated, elderly Irish man with late-stage

Alzheimer's disease. Arthur was referred for music therapy because he was isolated, spending most of the day puttering around his room, feeling confused. Despite his hearing loss, he responded to music, feeling the vibration of the drumbeat; he played along, creating much-needed social interaction.

One day, as our session started, his daughter and her husband arrived to visit. They were amazed to see how Arthur came alive through music, how he played the drum in perfect timing with me. I handed each of them a drum. Laughter filled the hall of the Alzheimer's unit as Arthur reached out with his drumstick and played everyone else's drum. Suddenly Arthur began to belt out an old Irish classic, "My Bonnie Lies over the Ocean." I looked over and saw that his daughter was beginning to cry. Tears rolled down her face, and I quietly asked whether she was OK. She nodded, bending over to share with me that her name was Bonnie, and her dad had named her after that song. Week after week, month after month, she had been visiting Arthur, despite the overwhelming sadness she felt when he did not recognize her. But that day, in the words of the song that was her namesake, she knew that somewhere in his heart, her father knew who she was.

Song Rehabilitation

When Arizona congresswoman Gabrielle Giffords survived a gunshot wound to the left hemisphere of her brain, a music therapist used singing to retrain her brain back to speaking.[21] Giffords's motivation came from the desire to sing "Happy Birthday" to her husband, as well as other favorite songs they both loved. Through singing, Gifford began to show improvement in speech. Love was the motivation.

Rehabilitation in song is called melodic intonation therapy (MIT). Melody is a well-established music-therapy tool of rehabilitation for stroke patients or for those with brain injuries that cause a loss of language skill. The effective use of melody in these patients shows that the left and right brain serve different functions in speech and song. This difference is why people who stutter can sing without problems, even as they struggle to talk. It works this way: we switch sides of our brains by changing speech into song, dancing around the brain damage and solidifying new neural pathways.

You may have heard the story of how country singer Mel Tillis's stuttering disappeared when he sang. Another example is the Oscar-winning movie *The King's Speech,* based on the true story of King George VI, whose speech impediment was rehabilitated by practicing his speeches in song.

Giving Song

Some songs may serve a future purpose that we do not yet know. We can carry a tune with us for years without knowing why. Giving song is the greatest heart gift; it is an act of the circuitry of music medicine. The giving-and-receiving cycle is healing for both singer and listener. Love is the key that always tunes our hearts.

Driving home on the Los Angeles freeway one rainy night, my teacher Uncle Manny Council Pipe Sandoval was suddenly hit by an oncoming car, causing his car to be totaled and his body to barely survive. When I went to see him in the hospital, I brought my drum and sat by his bed. Songs that Manny had taught me for Lakota ceremonies, prayers, and healing suddenly held new meaning. I felt as if I had learned them just for this moment, to sing them back to him.

As I sang a traditional welcoming song, I watched as his feet started to tap to the drumbeat. He began to softly mumble the melodies, even in his painful state. As I sang, he opened his eyes for the first time and tried to join my singing, as he continued to tap his feet along to the beat. The songs began to bring him back to life and brought me the compassion of giving that is the song of the heart.

Power Songs

In her book *The Four-Fold Way*, cultural anthropologist Angeles Arrien talks about power songs as a healing practice common among world indigenous traditions.[22] According to Arrien, power songs are an important source of strength, truth, and courage; they are also an empowerment tool associated with the visionary archetype. In a sense, songs help us hold the greater vision for ourselves and call in the intention to grow, heal, and bring our authentic voice into the world, the essence of melody.

We are intuitively drawn to the power songs we need. Sometimes songs find us. However it occurs, finding or recognizing your power song is important in the journey of music medicine. Sing your song regularly out loud or in your heart at times of need, or sing it as a regular practice of self-care.

For the past seven years, I've taught hundreds of people how to find and even write their own power songs. These songs serve as a personal anthem, much like a country's national anthem; they tell the story of great accomplishment and beauty. It's important to do more than affirm our good and to actually bring it to song. When I ask what songs people think of as power songs, I usually get answers like "I Will Survive," "I Believe I Can Fly," and "We Are the Champions." Notice the commonality of these songs? Notice the positive themes? Power songs are made of the best hopes, dreams, and truths set to melody so our hearts can resonate and remember their messages.

Song Synchronicity

Have you ever wondered how the perfect song comes on the radio or out of the shuffle function on your iPod just when you need it most? Or just when you miss someone, a song plays at the grocery store that makes you think of that person? Or a song comes on the radio reminding you of someone, and at that very moment, that person calls you? I call this *song synchronicity.*

We all have these stories of a song medicine moment. When I was thirty-five years old, my mother lost her two-year battle with stage IV ovarian cancer. After her passing, I went into a kind of hibernation in my own bereavement process, using many of the tools that I teach others for my own self-healing.

A month later, I was driving when the song "You've Got a Friend," sung by James Taylor, came on the radio, just when I was thinking of my mom. It was a song we sang to each other in the living room of her Cape Cod home a few months before she died. The synchronicity was uncanny. I felt as if she was sending me a message. Sometimes the universe is playing a radio station designed for healing moments for your heart.

Think of a time when song synchronicity graced the symphony of your life. Pay attention to what song pops into your life, and let yourself be with the magic that creates your own heart's healing. The next time you find yourself singing a tune for no reason at all, pay attention. Wonder about the song, its meaning, and its relevance in your life. It may have a deep message for you.

Heart Song

In his book of poems *Heartsongs,* Mattie Stepanek wrote that there is a song inside every person. Mattie was born with dysautonomic mitochondrial myopathy, a genetic condition that causes muscle, pulmonary, and cardiac problems. As the disease progressed, Mattie became wheelchair-bound and required oxygen. Nonetheless, he published five *New York Times* best-selling books. One of them, *Heartsongs,* was published when he was seven years old. Without any formal training or writing courses, his simple self-taught poetry expressed the song in his heart that wanted to be shared. Although he died at the age of twelve, the music of his heart lives on in his poetry.

In the title poem, Mattie wrote:

> *I have a song deep in my heart, and only I can hear it...*
> *It is so easy to listen to my song.*
> *If you believe in magical, musical hearts,*
> *you can be happy, then you, too, will hear your song.*[23]

What is stopping you from listening more deeply to your own heart song? Are you ready to bring more heart-centered melody into your life?

Final Chorus

Whether connecting to Spirit, family, nature, or our own inner voice, the medicine of melody is a sonic pathway to the heart. Melody is the medicine of emotional releasing, empowering, celebrating, remembering, and soothing our hearts. Melody is a medicine to empower our individual, authentic, unique voice. The medicine of melody is always singing in us, so we must listen, appreciate, and express its melody. We may stop singing but we can never lose our heart song. It can't be washed away.

GUIDED PRACTICES FOR
THE MEDICINE OF MELODY

These guided practices bring the healing medicine of melody into your heart and activate music's medicine as a tool for heart-centered living. Take a few moments to tune into your heart center. How does your heart need healing? Are you ready to live your life from your heart and to let your heart sing? What creates the happiness in you that makes your heart sing, and how can you bring more joy into your life? What needs soothing, awakening, or expressing?

In the process of both conscious listening and expressing, we attune ourselves to the songs that calm, restore, and heal our hearts. Explore these practices and follow what resonates with you. Add your own songs to the playlist and create your own heart's connection to the medicine of melody.

Guided Practices for Conscious Listening

Open Heart Listening
(Tracks 1, 3, 4, 10 from the online melody playlist)
Imagine that your heart has ears. Tune into melody that brings healing into the energy center of the heart. Start by listening to music without words, provided in the melody playlist. The absence of words allows you to more easily bypass the mind and move into the heart. Take a moment to consider what rich melodies have touched your heart. What sounds have called to your heart? Begin by tuning into your heart's preference.

When you're ready, take a moment to prepare to listen with the ears of your heart. Close your eyes and invite your heart to open. Place your hands over your heart or in any way that says your heart is listening. You can even cup your hand over your heart, in the way we cup our ears to indicate a more focused listening. Any way that feels right to you is best.

As the music begins, receive the melody in your heart. Let your heart be drenched in song. Let your heart ride the shape and motion of the notes, like surfing an ocean wave. Be open to hearing new things in the music— the heart has a way of feeling what the ears may not hear. If tears come up, allow them to be expressed and released. It may be an important release of something that has been weighing your heart for a long time. Give yourself permission to let it go. When the song is finished, allow a few moments of silence to let the benefits of the music sink into your whole self.

Listening to Spoken Song

When people speak, you can actually hear their melody. Attune your ears to the varying pitches and feeling tones communicated in a person's voice. You can hear the contrast between the voice of someone whose passion rings through every word spoken and the lifeless monotone of someone who is discouraged. Authenticity has a sonic equivalent. The truth is in the tone.

To attune to the melody hidden in speech, listen closely to the tune that underscores language, which is the prosodic aspect of speech. Hear the way the sonic melody of a question is different from that of a request. Try listening to the melody of someone's spoken voice. Can you hear the tune more than the word? Become conscious of your own voice. Notice how it sounds when you feel rested and restored, when talking about what you love, or after singing. Be aware of the words you speak as a tool of transmission of the melodic resonance of you.

Finding Your Power Song

Think of which songs have boosted your spirit, caused you to dance, or spoken a message that rings true in your heart. Our favorite songs are often our individual power songs. Our hearts have chosen them without realizing it. Take an inventory of powerful songs in your life. Power songs often appear in difficult and transitional times in our lives. Choose one power song that has meaning for your life right now. It may be a song that embodies the energy of some new goals you are trying to create or that helps empower your heart.

Make it a regular practice to consciously listen to or sing along with your power song. Adopt it as your personal anthem. Connect with the lyrics, melody, and energy. Find a good time of day to listen. It might be in the car on the drive to work, or it might be a way to start your day. If you feel so inspired, you can write your own power song by using a melody you already know but set to your own lyrics, or you can make up your own tune. It doesn't have to be long. What's important is putting it into practice in conscious listening.

Listening to Your Heart Song

The more you attune your heart to melody, the more you invoke a true song to call out from within you. This may happen naturally in an evolution of your own sonic awakening.

Take time to listen to your heart's melody. It may surprise you. It may be slower or faster than you'd expect. But one thing is consistent: your heart song is yours, unique in the entire world. To discover that heart song is to stand in your own authentic voice. Once you begin to hear it, hum along. Connect with your heart song throughout the day. Make it a practice to tuck your melody away deep within your heart in a place where no one else is listening. Notice how much your heart begins to resonate, feeling strong and melodious. Notice when you need to connect with your own heart. Sing your way back to heart.

Guided Practices for Expressing

Prana-Melodica

Before you begin to awaken your voice, start with proper breathing—the support system of breath that becomes song. I call it *prana-melodica*.

Many of us have never practiced breathing by using our diaphragm, the muscles that best support a strong vocal sound. Take a moment to simply put your hand on your belly and breathe. When you breathe into your diaphragm, your shoulders do not move; instead, your inhale should push your belly outward.

Diaphragm breathing is actually very natural; babies do it all the time. But as adults, we often have to retrain our bodies to breathe more deeply. To experience this, lie on your back in a prone position; your body will naturally use diaphragmatic breathing. Or try laughing. Those deep belly laughs naturally engage our diaphragm. So remember to use a strong, deep breath, a vital breath of life, for these melodic expression techniques. Trust that with a good breath, the sound will follow naturally.

Awaken Your Voice—Hum, Tone, Chant, Sing

(Tracks 4, 6, 7)

Here are four progressive steps toward melody, using the oldest instrument: the human voice. We move from the simple, accessible practice of humming, and follow into toning. Then we find chanting with the simple repetition of shorter phrases. And finally we move into full-on singing your heart out. Try these in a progression or find the one that resonates most with you.

1. *Humming.* Humming is a gentle way to warm up the voice and resonate different parts of the body by using low or high notes. When we hum, the lips are placed together and form the shape of a smile. Pick a note that is comfortable for you, and sustain the sound "mmmmmmm" or "hummmm." Close your eyes and feel the natural tingling. Vary the pitch and feel where the note resonates within your body. Can you sense a lower note moving down your throat into your heart center? Can you feel a higher note vibrating your forehead? Experiment and hum yourself awake.

2. *Toning.* Traditionally, toning is said to awaken energy centers in the body, including the heart. By simply sounding a single sustained note, you can resonate different energy centers of the body. Remember to take a deep prana-melodica belly breath before toning out loud. Since each person's body is different, it often takes a little noodling to find the pitch that resonates your heart and other energy centers. In some traditions, specific vowel sounds correlate with the body's energy centers. Often the sound "ahhhhhh" is connected to the heart tone. (Track 4 is a good example of vocalizing on the syllable "ah.") I've included other common associations of vowel sounds with energy centers, based on the work of Jonathan Goldman.[24]

Uh: Root

Ooo: Sacrum

Oh: Navel

Ah: Heart

I (pronounced "eye"): Throat

A (as in "hay"): Third Eye

Ee or Ohm: Crown

3. *Chanting.* Through the repetition of simple phrases, chants begin to encircle the heart. Sometimes, chanting the name of a person you wish to pray for can be a powerful form of healing. The practice of call-and-response devotional chanting is a good way to connect with the heart of spiritual practice. You can use the playlist recordings (tracks 6 and 7) or simply take a deep breath and repeat a short phrase or affirmation to your own melody.

4. *Singing.* Singing combines the expression of melody with lyrics that tell a heart's story. When your heart is awakened, you may catch yourself singing—in the shower, driving in the car, walking down the street. Find recordings of your favorite songs performed by an artist you resonate with, and sing along. It's good to find songs in your vocal range. Recall the creative spirit of the child within you that made up play songs; reconnect with your innate call to let your heart sing.

Heart Chant

(Track 8)
To connect with and embolden the radiance in your heart, you can listen to or chant along with the Heart Sutra, an ancient Buddhist scripture:

> *Om Gate Gate Paragate*
> *Parasamgate Bodhi Soha*

A *sutra* refers to a teaching or a line of thought that ties things together, similar to the term *sutures.* In the ancient language of Sanskrit, this mantra calls to the heart the perfection of transcendent wisdom. The Heart Sutra dates back to around 200–250 CE. The translation is "Gone, gone, gone beyond. Gone utterly beyond . . . Oh what an awakening!"

Sing along with the recording of the Heart Sutra from the melody playlist. Repetition is the key to allowing the chant to fall so deeply into your heart that you lose ego and time. Fall into your heart center in song.

Healing by Heart

To direct music medicine into your own heart center or into the heart space of someone else, play or sing a melody as an expression of healing by literally directing the sound to the heart. I call it playing to heart, as opposed to playing by heart. For example, I often use a Native American flute pointed at the person's heart center while I play an improvised melody that seems to express that person's heart sound. Because it's the melodic contour that shapes the heart, I vary the notes; I also use long tone mixed with shorter tone, and I include plenty of pauses. To see a video of this practice, visit youtube.com/ubdrumcircles.

This practice can be done for self-care or as a giving act of healing for another person's heart.

Self-care. You can use the melody of your own voice or a flute. When practicing for self-care, simply hold your hand over your heart and hum, tone, chant, or sing. Play the flute to bless the love in your heart.

Playing to another's heart. Begin by connecting with the person and setting an intention. Take a moment to become present to this practice of melody and healing. Using an instrument or your voice, begin by directing your sound into the person's heart. You might use a singing bowl, flute, thumb piano, or simply your voice. Perhaps sing the heart sound of "ahhhh." Trust your musical intuition and see what melodies come as a gift of heart.

ANNOTATED PLAYLIST FOR MELODY

To stream this music, visit SoundsTrue.com/MusicMedicine.

1. "Finding It Within," Nawang Khechog, *Sounds of Peace*
Listen deeply to this exquisite heart–opening melody of Nawang Khechog, Tibetan monk and Grammy-nominated musician, playing the Tibetan bamboo flute of his homeland.

2. "Medicine Melody 1," Silvia Nakkach, *Medicine Melodies*
Accompanied by the pan drum sound of the *hang,* Silvia Nakkach sings this piece. Nakkach is a music therapist, sound healer, author of *Free Your Voice,* and the founder of Vox Mundi (voxmundiproject.com). Listen to the way she sings a scale of unique contour as it carries you inside the notes of the scale. The music starts moving toward the end, getting the heart to dance.

3. "Inner Child," Dean and Dudley Evenson, *Sound Healing*
Joining the soft, gentle tones of the harp with a palette of bird songs and
nature sounds, the flute of Dean Evenson (of Soundings of the Planet)
reaches the heartstrings.

4. "Moon's Lament," Layne Redmond, *Invoking the Muse*
Sometimes the heart's song is a longing call—a releasing of pain, grief,
or deep desire for healing. Specifically sung to Melpomene, the muse of
singing, this recording joins flute and voice. Steve Gorn plays the *bansuri*
bamboo flute from India as women's voices chant the heart syllable "ah"
over the sweet groove of frame drums, *doumbek,* and *riq,* the
Egyptian tambourine.

5. "Shaman Journey," Silvia Nakkach, *Medicine Melodies*
Nakkach teams up with cellist David Darling for an improvisation on the
theme of heart healing, sung between the cello and voice over the soft
echoes of gongs and keyboards. Darling is also the founder of Music for
People (musicforpeople.org).

6. "Sita Ram," Jai Uttal, *Kirtan: The Art and Practice of Ecstatic Chant* Enter
the art of call-and-response devotional chant from the bhakti yoga tradition of India. Sita is the Infinite Goddess, the Divine Mother, and feminine
principle. Ram is the lord and masculine principle. Their love song is of the
divine couple, the union of male and female. Join Jai Uttal in this beautiful chant of the heart's love: "*Sita Ram Sita Ram Sita Ram Jay Sita Ram*"
(approximate translation: "Glory to Sita and Ram").

7. "Ahava Raba," YofiYah, *Kabbalah Kirtan*
Kirtan-style call-and-response singing with a song leader and choir is not
only done in the Sanskrit language from India. Artist YofiYah sings a heart-
filled call to the "great and magnificent Love." This morning liturgy is a
cultural perspective of the morning chant to greet the day. Sing along in
call-and-response style to the words "*Ahava Raba Ahavtanu,*" a Hebrew
phrase meaning "with great love You have loved us."

8. "Heart Sutra," Chloë Goodchild, *Fierce Wisdom*
This recording is for you to sing along. Make it a duet. Join the mantra or add your own voice in the rich spaces.

Om Gate Gate Paragate
Parasamgate Bodhi Soha

In the ancient language of Sanskrit, the heart mantra means "Gone, gone, gone beyond. Gone utterly beyond . . . Oh what an awakening!"

9. "Vorrei Vorrei," Priyo, *Gypsy Moon*
Vorrei is Italian for the calling out of the heart's desire, what it is you want. Let your heart dance to the gentle Afro-Mediterranean gypsy trance music of Priyo from Sicily, Italy. Let your heartstrings dance to the nylon string guitar. Let your heart be filled with song medicine.

10. "Giving and Forgiving," Nawang Khechog, *Quiet Mind*
Nawang Khechog plays the Tibetan flute in a lullaby to soothe your heart. The distinctive scale is filled with ornamented notes, rich pauses, and a sweet reverberation of the heart of peace.

5

Harmony: Medicine for the Soul

Let your soul be your pilot.
Let your soul guide you.
He'll guide you well.

—STING, "LET YOUR SOUL BE YOUR PILOT"

Harmony is the expression of the soul's desire for balance and connection. Just as melody helps us find our individual voice, harmony helps us discover the power of togetherness, our own inner sense of being "put together," and the bond created by harmonizing with other souls. Harmony creates a music bridge that transcends language, race, and cultural differences. As Rabindranath Tagore said, "Music fills the infinite between two souls."[1]

One rich moment of soul connection happened in Iraq when we were visiting the Institute of Kurdish Heritage, where we met the musicians and engineers who were preserving Kurdish cultural music common to northern Iraq. In the context of decades of oppression and genocide by Saddam Hussein's regime, Kurdish music became a symbol of national identity, a protected treasure that could not be captured or destroyed.

At the institute, I saw many instruments, but there was one in particular that fascinated me. It was a traditional Persian *tar*, the precursor of the *guitar*.

The tar is a peculiar-looking instrument with two circular soundboards covered with animal skin holding more than twenty strings. I learned that the instrument is tuned to quarter-tones in the ancient sound of the scales of the Far East—a sound that is foreign to most Western ears.

Spontaneously, a young man offered to play the tar for us. As I listened to his music, I was struck by his presence and generosity. When he finished playing, in an act of musical reciprocity, I pulled out my Native American cedar flute and played an improvised melody. I imagine the five-note scale of my flute sounded as foreign to his ears as the Kurdish scale did to mine.

Lydia, our translator, encouraged us to play together. I doubted it would work, considering that our scales were from such completely different cultures. I wondered if this could be the first time our two instruments—Persian guitar and Native American flute—were speaking to each other?

At first as we began to play together, it sounded out of tune. I tried to think about which notes could match between our different musical scales, but it was useless. Finally, I gave up and closed my eyes. The result was amazing. I began to hear the places where the pitches of our instruments came into harmony. We began to find each other in music, and a very surprising duet began to emerge. As we continued to play, the Iraqi musician adjusted his tuning, allowing us to weave our notes together and co-create music together. It was a powerful metaphor for how we must listen deeply to each other and make subtle tuning changes to be in harmony.

After the music came to a natural conclusion, I opened my eyes and felt an indescribable connection with the young man, created from soul-to-soul contact through the bridge of music. Smiles broke out on all the faces of the group gathered there that day to witness the unique duet—not just of the instruments, but also between two people who couldn't even speak the same language. We had found each other in the music and reached out across the sound barrier to bridge cultures in a harmony of souls.

Be in Harmony

We are incubated in rhythm and born in melody, and we grow and evolve in the harmony of relationships. We find harmony within ourselves in the balance of body, mind, and spirit, which are the three notes played together in a chord of wellness. Harmony is the nature of our souls. As Leonardo da Vinci said, "Don't you know the soul is composed of harmony?"[2]

We create harmony in relationships that enrich our souls, even calling the deepest, most intimate relationships "soul mates." Harmony and relationships require similar things: bending and blending, listening to each other, and adjusting our tuning as necessary. In harmony, something is created that is greater than any one instrument alone. In melody we create, and in harmony we co-create. Through harmony, we shift from "me" to "we" in the ensemble of interrelatedness. We need each other because the soul evolves through a symphony of support.

Harmony is embedded in our language of connection and togetherness. Living in peace and harmony refers to being in right relationship with people, animals, and nature. In music, chords are the basic building block of harmony. The word *chord* underscores our language of agreement; being of one accord, without which we have "dis-chord." When something resonates with our soul, we say it "strikes a chord."

Your soul's got music, and music's no good if it ain't got soul. The entire genre of music known as "soul music" has its origins in the rich, inspirational gospel singing. You may have experienced goose bumps while hearing the harmonies of a gospel choir. These harmonies bring out the soul, awakening that which is eternal in us all.

Lost Souls

Trauma and isolation create deep wounds in the soul. In traditional cultures, "soul retrieval" is the work of shamans, who use rituals based in sound and music to treat the underlying trauma that causes soul damage. Music's medicine in the form of chant and drumbeat creates the vibratory train ride to the spirit realms, where the shamans receive guidance and visions to locate missing pieces of the soul and bring them back. You might say that soul retrieval is essentially an act of reharmonizing.

What causes soul damage, and how prolific are these conditions? Experts identify trauma as a cause of soul damage—an emotional wound or shock that creates lasting psychological distress. Childhood abuse in the form of neglect, physical abuse, sexual abuse, and psychological maltreatment affects more than six million children annually. According to the U.S. National Child Abuse Statistics, a child abuse report is filed every ten seconds.[3] Those who survive the ravages of childhood abuse face greater challenges in soul recovery. Research shows that about 80 percent of individuals who were abused as children develop at least one psychological disorder, indicating a proliferation of soul damage.[4]

When I worked as a social worker and music therapist in foster care, I treated children with attachment disorder, a condition caused by a lack of bonding with parents at an early age that leads to lack of trust and a resistance to forming relationships. I saw the deep soul damage caused by the cycle of abuse that repeats from generation to generation. To heal this damage, I created group music experiences to increase bonding between foster children and their adoptive parents. Music creates easier access to a child's soul than does talking. The approach was effective, particularly because of the natural laws of harmony. No one wants to make bad music together; there was an intrinsic motivation toward finding a good sound together, and this motivation created musical bonding that transferred into soul-level healing and more openness to trust.

Trauma rises in times of war, causing damage to soldiers, families, and whole nations. Current statistics estimate that 20 percent of the 1.6 million men and women who have served in Iraq and Afghanistan have Post-Traumatic Stress Disorder (PTSD). In 2005, the U.S. Department of Veterans Affairs (VA) indicated that PTSD was the fourth most common service-related disability for service members receiving benefits.[5] Forced to be constantly on guard and witnessing acts of violence, soldiers often find the adjustment to civilian life when they return from the battlefield to be difficult.

Recent research has illuminated actual brain changes caused by trauma, including flooding of emotional centers, hypersensitivity of the fight-or-flight response, and extreme startle responses caused by auditory and visual triggers. The physical self may be back home, but parts of the soul may remain in the battlefield.

When I returned to the United States from our drum-circle project in Iraq, I spoke at a conference attended by counselors who were treating returning American soldiers, the "wounded warriors." As we shared our observations, we realized the remarkable similarities between the challenge of treating American veterans and my experience working with Kurdish survivors of genocide. It gave me an awareness that no one wins in war. No matter which side you are on, the soul damage that is suffered is prolific.

Another factor causing soul damage is a sense of being disconnected. Whether due to trauma or a loss of community, loneliness is on the rise. A recent survey showed that more than one-third of American adults reported feeling lonely.[6] Over a period of almost fifty years, the number of Americans living alone more than doubled, up from 10 percent in 1950 to 24 percent in 1994. The rate is shockingly higher in seniors, our soul-blood of wisdom, with 40 percent of those over age seventy-five living alone.[7]

The opposite can be true as well. We can become deprived of the solitary time needed to tune into our soul. Patterns of overcommitment, being too busy, or tending to the needs of others more than ourselves pull us away from our soul's song. When we take time to listen to our soul, we hear our purpose and create its expression in our life, aided by the support of community.

Have you taken time to tune into your soul? Do you know what helps you connect with your soul? Is your life in harmony with your soul's purpose? Are you able to connect with others and create the rich harmony that nurtures your soul?

There is another cause of soul damage, a condition of our fast-paced world of ever-accelerating technology. We may be moving so fast that we leave our souls behind. There is a story of the first train ride taken by Native American railroad workers, which was told to me by Mark Makai. It is said that the handful of Native American men were leery of the train's speed compared with their familiar pace traveling by horse. Initially they refused to ride the train, but eventually they were persuaded to do so. After an hour, the train made a short stop, allowing the passengers to get off for a while. The Native American men slowly strode off the train and sat under the shade of a tree. When the train whistle blew, everyone else scurried back to the train, but they didn't move. When the conductor came out, he asked them, "What are you doing just sitting there? Don't you hear it's time to go?" The men simply replied, "We are waiting for our souls to catch up."

The Art of Harmony

Harmony is defined as the "relationships between notes" and "the pleasing combination of differences." The natural world is built on harmony—the interplay of different pollinators and plants, the movement of schools of fish flowing with the ocean's currents, the duet of rivers joining and flowing to the sea. Seasons change, storms come and go, but the soul of nature keeps singing. The universe operates in harmony, which Greek mathematician and philosopher Pythagoras called the harmony of the spheres—or the way the universe is held together in balance, yet is moving and expanding in a symphony of science.

Life Wants to Harmonize

There is a natural force of harmony that wants to be in balance. In musical language, it's called *consonance*. When we make music together, the law of harmony pulls our notes naturally into the simple intervals of beauty.

Pygmies in Africa join together in an exquisite harmony of different voices matching and reflecting the sonic landscape of nightfall in a forest, where crickets play a different part than frogs, woven with coyote howls, wind whistling, and streams babbling. Tribal cultures living close to nature have demonstrated the force of harmony for centuries.

The Four Agreements of Harmony

In harmony, as in life, playing together requires agreements that create the shared space for co-creating. From the smallest ensemble of a duet or trio to choirs, orchestras, and symphonies, group music making requires being in tune, playing in the same key, keeping together in the same rhythm, and following the same chord progression. These parts are often indicated on a musical score or discussed before a jam begins.

In music's medicine, we move through four stages as we harmonize. I call these the four agreements of harmony. You'll recognize the parallel between music and life.

1. *Be in Tune.* Like any music ensemble, before we can play together, we have to be in tune, which requires listening to ourselves first. Being in tune allows us to connect to the instruments in life's ensemble. Tuning is ongoing throughout the harmonizing process.

2. *Join In.* We share a common pace and pulse of the rhythm, as well as a common key and tonality of the composition. In music, we unite through the common agreements of the key and rhythm. What is the tonality of the key, the pace, and pulse of the rhythm? In life, we match and support others to strengthen our common song.

3. *Blend In.* We harmonize by bending and blending and creating an interplay between ourselves and the ensemble. Dynamics guide our volume, tuning in to whether we need to play down or amplify in order to best contribute. We listen for what's missing in the note or rhythm of the ensemble and add what's needed. In life, we practice the art of bringing our unique notes into the ensemble of our relationships and communities.

4. *Co-create.* At its most creative stage, harmony is a co-creation in which no one is leading. When we co-create in harmony, we discover a shared muse that is the basis of creativity between players. When you get off the sheet of written music and into the process of improvisation, magic emerges. The force of harmony and creativity guides the music. Everyone is contributing, and no one is dominating. Everyone owns co-created harmony. It's a healing force for peacemaking and a model for human empowerment. When we trust the process and invest our souls, harmony takes us to newly invented music that is greater than anyone can imagine. Beauty is our natural outcome.

The Progression of the Soul

As our souls evolve, our notes change and affect our relationships. In music, harmonic intervals—the distance between two simultaneous notes—behave like relationships in life.

An interval can be consonant or dissonant, close or distant. Our ears recognize when things sound good or are out of tune, just as our souls recognize the harmony or dissonance in relationships. If one person in a relationship changes pitch or vibration, suddenly the "old way" of being together changes and becomes temporarily dissonant.

In music, dissonance begs to be resolved. When it is resolved, tension is released. Notice the places where the notes of your relationships have changed, whether they are your notes or another person's. Listen for the resolution that is naturally inherent in the drive for harmony.

Jazz musicians call the harmonic motion of music the *progression.* Like music, our souls are here to evolve, to progress. Each chord, each relationship, each trio and quartet of notes in our lives comes together and resonates a specific tonality; it may be bright and open like a major chord, or it may be somber and inward like a minor chord. Listen to the tonality of the different chords at play in the progression of your life. Even the dissonant ones may be an important part of the progression.

The Principle of Harmony—Sympathetic Vibration

There is real meaning behind the idea that something can "strike a chord" in us. In psychoacoustics, the principle of sympathetic vibration, or sympathetic resonance, shows that when a single string is played, the same string on a separate instrument will actually sound without being struck. For example, placing two guitars side by side and playing the bottom string on only one guitar will vibrate the same string on the second guitar, even though it was not physically touched. Instruments resonate with each other; their sound frequencies harmonize and amplify. It is the resonance between instruments that creates the potential for sympathetic activation.[8]

Sympathetic vibration not only creates sound in another instrument, it can also be felt kinesthetically. In drum circles, I often invite half the group to place their hands on their drums and feel the vibration of the rest of the group playing. People break into smiles of amazement as they feel the beat coming through the drum and pulsing in their resting hands. In this sense, there can be no unplayed drums in a drum circle.

Scientific evidence shows that sympathetic vibration goes well beyond the principle of harmony—it is also mirrored in our human interactions. Like instruments, we are affected by the vibrations of those around us, and we are equally effective in resonating others. Empathy, compassion, and a greater awareness of our impact on one another are all keys to the living practice of the medicine of harmony.

The Shadow Side of Harmony

There can be self-created barriers to nature's laws of harmony. Some people lack experience in the art of human harmonizing. Dissonance is a disease of those who create conflict to avoid deeper emotions, pain, and loss. When our souls are out of tune, we find that the chords of life have changed, sometimes sounding dissonant. We may be on the receiving side of a work colleague or loved one who has changed his or her tune. For example, you may face a difficult boss who is out of tune, upset, and angry. The note he or she communicates is one of blame and frustration. It's difficult to harmonize as the interval between the two of you becomes dissonant. In extreme cases, the lack of harmony can lead to war and violence.

Cultural differences in our upbringing also affect our harmonizing. In Asian cultures, the needs of the family and community take precedence over the needs of the individual. By contrast, much of the Western world's prioritization focuses on the individual. Regardless of our cultural upbringing, we can choose whether we are about the "me" or the "we," and we can then move toward a balance of both aspects—calibrated and in concert.

Resolution is a natural *soul*ution for dissonance. *Resolution* is a term that applies to conflict resolution as much as it does to musical resolution; it means there is a dissonant chord that begs to move toward consonance. Harmonic motion can carry us toward consonance if we allow it to move us and move through us.

The Science of Harmony

From wave frequencies resonating an unstruck chord to our human neural wiring, which fires in mirroring patterns of empathy, harmonizing is woven into the science of humanity. Once again, science is documenting how we are innately wired for harmony and how important feeling connected is for our health and our souls.

Wired for Resonance

In the past twenty years, researchers have identified a set of neurons referred to as "mirror neurons," which perform much like the principle of sympathetic vibration. Simply watching the actions of another person resonates these neurons. Even when we are only observing, parts of our brains respond as if we were performing the same action that we witnessed. The existence of mirror neurons has given scientists insights into how we are wired for compassion and empathy—qualities that develop our souls.

In experiments in which subjects watch a film of a person falling down and hurting the right knee, the subjects' brains lit up in areas matching the experience of right knee pain. When we see a strong emotional or physical occurrence of someone else, we literally feel that person's pain.[9] However, it's not only watching an action that causes these neurons to fire. Studies reveal that even hearing a sound associated with an action can trigger our brain's sympathetic mirror reaction.

Christian Keysers, PhD, of the Social Brain Lab in the Netherlands, tested monkeys by using the sounds of specific actions: ripping paper, breaking a peanut, or dropping a stick. He found that the neurons in the observing monkeys fired as if they themselves were performing the tasks that matched the sounds.[10] Mirror neurons were ignited in about 20 percent of the whole brain area that would function when performing the corresponding action.

Extending his research into humans, Keysers found similar sympathetic neural firing upon both seeing and hearing action tasks. The subjects who were shown a picture of a face expressing disgust or who heard the sounds associated with that feeling had mirror activation of similar areas in their brains. They literally felt what others were feeling.[11]

Neurons of Harmony

If you've ever felt captivated by watching the graceful rhythmicity of a conductor in an orchestra, you may not be surprised to hear that new research is beginning to pinpoint how live music engages our souls. Researchers are finding that it's the musical gestures—hand movements, conducting, the way an instrument is played, and even facial expressions when singing—that resonate with the mirror neurons in our brains.

Istvan Molnar-Szakacs, PhD, of the University of California, Los Angeles, and Katie Overy, PhD, of the Institute for Music in Human and Social Development in Edinburgh, Scotland, developed a theory of the role of mirror neurons in how we are moved by music. The key is in the movement used in performing music and the emotional expressions of musical communication. They found that even watching musical gestures excites mirror neurons in the motor and emotional brain, as if we were actually performing. According to their study, mirror neurons in both motor and emotional brain areas work together to translate musical gestures into a sympathetic response.[12] It could be music's motion that becomes the emotion that moves our souls.[13] This explains how musicians who are more overtly expressive when they perform move us more so than do less expressive performers. You can truly sense when someone is putting more soul into music.

Banding Together

Moving from neuroscience to social science, we discover evidence of the healing benefits of social activities in which we harmonize with others.

When Robert Putnam published his book *Bowling Alone,* he launched the use of *social capital* as an umbrella term for the interdisciplinary study of social networks, social connection, and civic participation.[14] Based on large survey results, his research demonstrated that building our social capital through participation in group activities translates to more happiness, health, and sense of purpose in life. Put simply, the more social capital we create, the less isolation and the greater benefits we experience, not only in physical health but also in our state of mind and state of soul.

Soul research looks at outcome measures that track body, mind, and spirit in concert, collectively referred to as "quality of life." This quality of life includes the spiritual, physical, emotional, and social aspects of well-being. Thus, the richer the activation of the soul, the stronger the quality of life.

Participation in a choir is one of the most common forms of harmonizing. According to the 2009 Chorus Impact Study, 18 percent of households reported at least one adult who belongs to a choir, and 32.5 million adults reported regularly singing in choruses.[15] The report also found that the harmonious benefits of belonging to a chorus extend into life. Choral members become better team players and are more socially compassionate. They volunteer more and demonstrate increased community involvement with a more positive attitude. Their souls are evolving in a positive progression.

Stephen Clift at the Research Center on Arts and Health in Canterbury, England, performed one of the largest studies on choral singing to date. With more than one thousand choristers from three countries—Germany, the United Kingdom, and Australia—Clift used the World Health Organization's holistic health assessment to track the quality of life of the singers. Although half the choristers, whose average age was fifty-seven, reported significant health challenges, a remarkable 87 percent still rated their health as very good to excellent. This rating was much higher than a matched control group who did not sing in a choir. Belonging to the choir seemed to improve the singers' perception of their health.[16]

In a follow-up study delving more deeply into the subjects' perceptions of the effect of choir to overcome their challenges, Clift identified key activation/deactivation patterns that are specific on/off switches operated by the experience of harmony. Again, it's not only what music *does* for the soul but also what it *undoes.* I've summarized Clift's findings in the areas of mind, body, spirit, and social bonding.

1. *Mind*. Focusing attention and engaging the mind in choir switches off preoccupation with worry and reduces cognitive decline, which is associated with aging.

2. *Body*. The deep-controlled breathing involved in singing provides a motivation for exercise and decreases resistance to physical activity.

3. *Spirit*. The positive effect felt in choir and the sense of support found in singing together decrease loneliness, sadness, anxiety, and depression.

4. *Social*. Belonging to the group and participating in regular rehearsals decrease inactivity, isolation, and social disengagement.

Like choirs, bands demonstrate improvement in soul-filled qualities of life. A study showed that the New Horizons Band Program for seniors developed group identity; created a sense of belonging; and built a strong sense of reciprocity, trust, commitment, and compassion for each other. New bridges were formed between people who would never have met otherwise. In addition, performances and service opportunities in the broader community connected people who would not ordinarily engage with each other.[17] For more information about New Horizons Band, visit newhorizonsmusic.org.

There is a growing trend of less-formal music groups, which may be necessary, given our soul's need for nourishment and awakening. The whole movement of amateur music participation, called "recreational music making," is defined by the National Association of Music Merchants as group participation in music experiences for health and well-being. According to Kala Brand Ukuleles, more than one thousand ukulele clubs have sprung up worldwide in the past five years. Drum circles are also on the rise, forming in parks, schools, hospitals, and churches and are being led by thousands of trained drum-circle facilitators.

Happiness: The Soul's Longing

A common note resounds as to why we harmonize: happiness. This could be the main scientific outcome of a fully expressed, connected, empowered soul. In one study, 85 percent of choir members agreed with the statement "singing has made me a happier person." Happiness outperformed other choices, such as feeling good after a performance (70 percent) or releasing negative thoughts or feelings (66 percent). It seems that nothing beats a soul in harmony.[18] In the New Horizons Band study, subjects reported that the bonds between band members in soul-felt relationships were most responsible for their happiness. In fact, the relationships created through harmonizing scored even higher than improved health and reduced pain and medical problems in terms of what most contributed to band members' happiness.[19]

In summary, the principle of sympathetic vibration between instruments seems to be similar to the sympathetic mirroring neuron systems in animals and humans alike. Compassion, empathy, and sympathy arise through the harmonic experience of seeing and hearing actions that move the soul. When we step across the threshold from watching performers into co-creating music together, in ensembles of singing or playing instruments, we experience the sense of belonging that is the medicine of harmony. The conclusion is this: we are wired to harmonize.

The Spirit of Harmony

Music's medicine of harmony is a universal practice born of our soul's longing for union, which transcends cultures and religions. According to many traditions, the soul is the eternal point within us all. Whether it is the exquisite duet of our individual soul with the Creator or an ensemble of music makers, through harmony, we feel each other's souls.

When the Dalai Lama spoke at the World Festival of Sacred Music in Los Angeles in 1999, he said, "Music symbolizes the yearning for harmony—within oneself, with others, with nature, and with the spiritual and sacred within us and around us. There is something in music which transcends and unites."[20]

According to the Gospel of Matthew (18:20), Jesus says, "For where two or three come together in my name, there am I with them."[21] In an interpretation of the teachings of Jesus by Mary Magdalene, a similar message of harmony is clear: "To be in harmony is to be in a conscious and loving relationship with what is. Harmony means to have a musical relationship with the world, to enter into resonance, to be in tune with all that is."[22] Put simply, the spirituality of harmony is becoming calibrated and in concert.

Nature is constantly revealing the spiritual principle of harmony. It is up to our awareness to recognize its song. Both Shinto and Buddhist traditions value the way nature demonstrates the spirit of harmony. Temple grounds are filled with exquisite Zen gardens, which are a statement of natural harmony, referred to in the phrase *wabi-sabi*. To use a metaphor of music, wabi-sabi is the recognition of nature singing in perfect harmony. Perhaps it's the way a vine reaches around a neighboring branch or the way cypress trees form an inviting grove. It could be a small crop of mushrooms growing from rich moss or the spiritual practice of sculpting a bonsai tree, balancing its many branches in a harmonious effect.

The Music Bridge

Harmony is a spiritual bridge linking two souls. I call it the music bridge. Like a bridge from one side of a river to the other bank, all that separates us symbolically can be crossed in the shared experience of harmony. Bridges on guitars have a similar function. Strings rest upon the bridge to be amplified and transmitted throughout the rest of the instrument and then into the world.

If you've ever experienced humming along to the wind, tapping to the rhythm of the rain, or howling in response to coyotes at dusk, you know the feeling of connecting with the soul of nature in sound. Likewise, you feel the soul-to-soul communion in life when you harmonize by singing or making music with someone else. If you dare to hold eye contact while the music is happening, the experience of soul connection is even more profound.

Perhaps the greatest experience of being in harmony is union with the Divine Presence, the Creator, or as *The Radiance Sutras* say, the Great Musician. To illustrate this concept with a music metaphor, I think of my connection to Spirit as being two notes with a bar line bridging them together. The bar line symbolizes how we are not separate from the Divine Presence, which is a slightly higher note. Even the term *yoga* refers to the "yoke," or the bridge between oxen, which symbolizes the link between ourselves and the sacred. In music, this is the bar line. Our souls thrive in the experience of this divine duet, harmonizing with the presence of the Creator in our lives, in our souls, and in all aspects of life's rich music. In my representation of this idea, I include wings around the notes to represent the lightness, flight, and freedom in moments of music communion between our souls and the soul of Spirit.

Instruments of Harmony

From the vocal chords singing to the strumming of guitars, the soul is reached in chords, like the heart is with strings. Angels are often depicted playing lutes, precursors to the guitar that date back to the seventh century CE. Pianos, organs, and guitars are other chord-making instruments that appear in sacred spaces. Ethnomusicologists call these instruments *chordophones.* Saint Cecilia, the Catholic patron saint of music, is often depicted playing a piano, with light streaming upon her hands. Organs have long been associated with church music; a small, portable organ called the *harmonium,* named for harmony, is used in India and worldwide for devotional chanting. In Mexico, mariachi bands of guitars play music to accompany church congregations singing together.

In world cultures, the individual instruments that make up an ensemble are built and referred to as a family. In West African drumming, the three low-pitched drums are referred to as mother, father, and child. Balinese *gamelan* music is played on a set of metallic percussion instruments that are built and tuned to each other. The tuning is specific to each ensemble such that you can't remove one instrument and go play with another group. The instruments are themselves a family, tuned and harmonized in relation to one another. What a great metaphor for life. We are all instruments of harmony.

Saraswati's Guitar

Saraswati, the Hindu goddess of knowledge, wisdom, and the audible arts, plays the *vina,* a seven-string Indian guitar. I think of her as a deity of harmony. She is said to have originated from a river, reminding us of the watery flow of harmonic motion. In harmony, notes, like rivers and tributaries, flow together and coalesce into chords. Benzaiten, the Japanese version of Saraswati, holds a *shamisen,* a Japanese guitar. Saraswati's music symbolizes the spiritual path of living in perfect harmony with the world.

Gospel Music

Years ago, the sound of gospel singing coming from a church near my apartment in upstate New York drew me into a Pentecostal church called the Soul Saving Station for Every Nation, based in Harlem. Drawn in by the sounds of rich harmonies accompanied by a Hammond B-3 organ, I entered the church. Although

I was in the minority, I spent the next year covered in goose bumps as the Gospel choir sang and the grandmothers played tambourines while dancing in the aisles or seated in the pews. Somehow word spread that I was a musician, and soon I was filling in on drums and piano when the regular players were absent. Imagine, a white girl playing with a black gospel ensemble. It was quite a sight.

Due to an unfortunate battle with cancer, the regular organist became ill and had to resign. Pastor Byrd said, "Sister Christine, God told me you would play the organ now." I was shocked because I did not know how to play the organ, but how can you turn down a call from God? The call to serve reaches the soul.

The next week, many of the revered mothers and grandmothers of the church joined the pastor in a ceremony to prepare me to play the organ. They gathered around me while Pastor Byrd anointed my hands with oil. For the entire ensuing year, I played organ, accompanying the music that had drawn me into this powerful spiritual tradition. In harmony, I discovered my colorless soul and became part of the ensemble. As much as I was drawn in by the harmony, it ended up drawing more music out of me. I was able to experience the law of harmony—giving back to the music that had fed my soul.

Communion of Saints

In musical harmony, we move from verbal communication to soul communion. I once led a large drum circle with a group of more than one hundred Methodist ministers at a conference in the mountains of Colorado. Joined by my colleague Jon Crowder, of Peak Rhythms, we brought together spiritual chant and communal rhythms in a powerful experience that inspired one woman to claim, "This was like the communion of Saints." To see a video of the Methodist minister drum circle, visit youtube.com/ubdrumcircles.

Throughout my worldwide work in places of language barriers, I have found one resonant truth: words communicate thoughts, but music communicates energy. During our work in Iraq, I was inspired by a moment of generosity in the final performance of our drum-circle training, which was attended by more than one hundred community members, government officials, and even the First Lady of Iraq, Mrs. Hero Talibani. Toward the end of the performance, without my direction, the group we had trained walked into the audience and offered their drums, begging others to join the drum circle. Harmony creates generosity.

All My Relations

In Lakota sacred teachings, we are all related. Even newcomers to a ceremony are welcomed with "Hello, Relatives." Living in harmony in right relationships with all living things is the basis of life. Everything is treated with deep respect and honoring, including people, animals, and all of nature. Imagine the harmony that could exist on the planet if we were all to recognize how interrelated we are? *Mitakuye oyasin* in Lakota Sioux means "all my relations," a phrase that embodies this belief and that often begins and ends prayers. The sacred hoop is held as a symbol of uniting the four races—the white, red, black, and yellow people of the world. Ceremonies act out the return of the harmony of humanity and the oneness of living as relatives with all things by bringing all the colors, and the races, together into the wheel.

In learning the Lakota language through singing and attending ceremonies, I've developed a better understanding of this cosmology of connection. The belief of interconnectedness is present in words like *oyate* (o-ya-tay), meaning "the nation." An individual tree is referred to as the "tree nation"; a stalk of sage as the "sage nation." In this way, we are all part of the "music nation."

The practice of living in harmony is evident in the Lakota way of balance between giving and receiving, an ever-present awareness of the harmony of exchange. When sage is picked for a ceremony, tobacco is given to the sage nation in gratitude. Songs are chanted to thank the life of herbs, trees, and stones. Nothing is taken without giving back to the source of its medicine.

The Medicine of Harmony—Ensemble Medicine

If you have ever played in a band, sung in a choir, or belonged to a music group, you've been touched by ensemble medicine. An *ensemble* is defined as "many elements coming together for one desired effect." Choirs breathe together, orchestras count measures in unison, and drum ensembles pulse at the same time as dancers in village rituals. World cultures understand ensemble medicine and invite everyone to join the singing, playing, and dancing of community rituals. I consider the harmony of community and ceremony to be medicine for the soul's unfolding, healing, and revealing. Harmony draws us into connection.

What can we learn from cultures that emphasize community over individuality? What is the healing benefit of this way of living for the soul? When I traveled to Asia to teach drum circles for health and wellness, I immediately sensed the difference in cultural ways of thinking. Japanese culture was more focused on family, community, and togetherness, making me aware of my Western individualism. The contrast was audible in the way Japanese people played together in the drum circle. In America, I had to work to get a group to listen to each other in drum circles. I was shocked in Japan, and in many other parts of Asia, when everyone played easily in unison. The cultural emphasis on "we" versus "I" brought a benefit to the drumming.

However, when I invited the group to add more individual expression and make up their own music, there was confusion. My request seemed to be lost in translation. I eventually demonstrated the individuality of improvisation, and the drum-circle participants slowly began to take more and more risks and add their own rhythms to the unified groove.

Similarly, working in Iraq, the sense of community focus was apparent in the typical way of dancing. Kurdish and Arab dances involve linking arms and moving together in line dances or circles. What a contrast to my Western way of free-dancing alone. Their dancing style was even greater than the typical partner dance—it was communal dance.

At first, joining in the Japanese rhythms or Kurdish dances felt restrictive to me, but this was a small price to pay for the eventual feeling of being part of the whole. I sensed the power of the healing force that was inherent in the feeling of togetherness.

Ensembles of Empowerment

Bringing the medicine of harmony to corporate America has been a large part of my work in the past decade. I call it harmonizing; they call it team building. Companies are often filled with different *divisions,* a term that, in itself, can lead to a misinterpretation of the challenge in working as a team. As in the definition of *ensemble,* a company strives to come together for one desired effect embodied in the mission statement or corporate goals. In the metaphor of music, teams experience making music together, harmonizing divisions and different parts that weave together to create one groove.

Families can benefit from ensemble medicine as well. When I worked with foster children and their biological parents, I used instruments to assess and bring ensemble medicine into families. I brought drums and shakers of varying power and size, and began with an open invitation for family members to choose what they wanted to play. The child who was taking on a parenting role would choose the loudest drum, while the absent parent would choose a soft shaker. It gave me an accurate assessment of the family's power differentials. Then I asked everyone to change instruments, symbolizing taking on new roles by literally playing a new part in the family ensemble. As I orchestrated the new music, we could discuss the shifting sound of more functional family roles. A new ensemble emerged.

Soul Tending

Togetherness is a healing force, a medicine of harmony that creates a sense of belonging and offers soul-to-soul connection when we feel alone. There are times in life's difficult journeys when the soul is damaged, lost, or devastated. Sometimes we have no control over the circumstances in our lives. Especially in these scenarios, having a sense of support from someone who brings a healing vibration into our lives is part of the reharmonizing of our souls. It may even be an animal that helps create the union of soul healing.

Just like musical relationships, healing relationships take many forms. Perhaps it is a duet of working with a therapist, partner, family member, or soul friend. Or maybe it is a healing trio when three join together, quartets in four, quintets in five, and larger ensembles of support groups. One of the great principles of success in Alcoholics Anonymous is the sense of harmony between members in a meeting. Without hierarchy, the sense of support and inclusivity, as well as the assignment of sponsors who give back based on what they have received, is all part of the program's extraordinary success. It's not unlike the Lakota practice of living in harmony with all our relations.

A Duet of Healing

Harmony refers to "different notes coming together," but what if the differences in the notes are extreme, as in the case of actual enemies? Can music really create change, even when the notes are in conflict?

When I was working in Iraq, our Kurdish translator was a young man in his early thirties named Shalo. Like most Kurds, his father had fought against Saddam Hussein's oppression for more than a decade, disappearing for months at a time into the mountains. Shalo still remembered his fear that his father would never come home while the family was hiding in the mountains during the 1991 Kurdish exodus. After the American liberation, Shalo got his father back, but life was forever changed.

I wondered how Shalo felt being in the drum circle with Arabs. Their fathers had probably fought against each other. To make it even more interesting, one of the training participants was from Tikrit, Saddam Hussein's hometown. I wondered how the obvious tension would play out.

One day during a break in the training, I heard music echoing down the hall. I followed the sound to a small room, where Shalo was playing violin with the Arab drummer from Tikrit. Here they were, creating a duet in the very space where torture had occurred less than a decade ago. I waited outside the room, hidden away, moved by my awareness of the meaning of this musical exchange. When the music naturally finished, the men emerged from the room. They had entered as Kurd and Arab, yet they left the room as an ensemble, playing together in harmony.

In the next few days, I noticed the two men hanging out together on breaks. There was a continuation of the musical bonding. At the end of the training, Shalo was visibly moved by his experience. What had begun as a routine job as a translator became the transformation of the soul through the power of harmony. "I never thought I could have a friend from Tikrit," he told us. "We learned to make music together; we learned how to work in peace together." He told us he had exchanged e-mail addresses with his new friend, and they hoped to stay in contact. When you make music together, you can no longer be enemies.

Final Chorus

Harmony is what our souls are made of. Our soul evolves in the sharing of harmonic relationship with all living things. It calibrates our souls. Not surprisingly, the principle of sympathetic vibration reminds us how we are all affected by each other, a finding rooted in scientific evidence of our neurology of empathy and mirror neuron system. World cultures that live and practice harmonizing with nature and one another remind us that we are all related. Harmony invites us to join the community, deepen trust, and build relationships. In the words of Lao-tzu, "Music in the soul can be heard by the universe."[23]

GUIDED PRACTICES FOR THE MEDICINE OF HARMONY

These practices have been developed to support you in bringing harmony into the places in your life where it's missing. Take a few moments to tune into your soul. Where in your life do you need greater soul expression, soul connection, and harmony?

The first set of practices focuses on conscious listening with the ears of the soul, developing greater harmonic awareness, and listening to your soul song. The second set of practices shows you how to express your soul through harmony, to create duets and dialogues with other souls and the elements of nature, and ultimately to resonate with the chords of life.

Guided Practices for Conscious Listening

Listen to Your Soul Song

(All tracks from the harmony playlist)

Using the harmony playlist, you can practice receiving the medicine of harmony in your soul listening. You may also have songs that have touched your soul, given you goose bumps, or taken you into the realm of the eternal. It may be an *a capella* choir, rhythm and blues, gospel, or a church hymn. What sounds call to your soul? Add them to your playlist.

When you are ready for some soul listening, take a moment to dedicate your practice to an area of your life that needs more harmony or a place in your soul that needs greater expression. Take a breath and feel into your soul. Close your eyes and sense the part of you that is eternal. Make a physical statement of where you feel your soul—perhaps encircling you, or perhaps deep within you? Or perhaps both?

As you prepare to listen to the music, let go of your body awareness. Become one with the full richness of the music. Listen from a place beyond the body. Drink it up in the depths of your soul. Maintain a wide focus, like a multidirectional microphone of your soul. Listen like an owl that spins its head and turns its ears all around. Develop harmonic awareness to music. Listen to the motion of the whole ensemble. Notice the starting key and the progression throughout the music, the movement away from and returning to the original key. Let the sympathetic strings of your soul resonate with the music's harmony.

Harmonic Awareness

Harmonic awareness is a practice that focuses on the relationship between elements more than on their separateness. You can practice harmonic awareness by sitting in nature. Take time to be in a favorite outdoor place and hear with the ears of the soul the composition created by nature. It is always new, never the same, never repeated. Listen for the relationships between sounds, rather than listening for separate sounds. Hear dialogues and duets between birds or between the crickets or frogs at nightfall. Hear the rhythm of leaves rustling in the wind while a stream babbles running over rocks. Let your soul enjoy this time of harmony.

Extend your harmonic awareness to the flow of life. Where in your life do you notice the harmony, a natural blending or togetherness, the sense of being in right relationship? Notice moments of harmony between yourself and others, movements of shared rhythms that allow a matching and collaboration to occur. Explore how effortless it is to live within the law of how life wants to harmonize. Pay attention to the music of life and join the ensemble.

Ensemble Ears

This practice can change how you perceive and receive live music. Even in spiritual services, live music often accompanies the gathering. Bring a soulful awareness to listening to the band or choir. At any live music performance or event, notice the way the band members interact. Absorb how they work together, play off each other, breathe together, and blend. If you like jazz, go watch a jazz ensemble and notice the improvisation that ebbs and flows in waves of harmonies. Jazz ensembles play off each other and build upon each other's creativity. You will feel and hear the flow of the progression like ocean waves that build energy, crest, and then rescind. Take yourself out on a soul date of harmony.

Soul Music Sharing

Create a shared practice of listening together with a loved one to develop greater intimacy between your souls. This is a great practice to do with a soul mate. Choose music that you love, that stirs your soul. Invite your partner to bring his or her music, be it a short playlist or a full CD by a favorite artist. Turn off all distractions—cell phones, e-mails, and computers—and give each other's music your full soul attention.

A music bridge is created in shared listening that allows a connection of souls. What can you learn about another's soul from his or her musical selection? What do you reveal about yours? Take turns listening together and honor a silent pause between each piece.

Guided Practices for Expressing

Play a Duet with Nature

(Track 4)

Go into your favorite place in nature, where you feel a sense of harmony. Let your soul listen. From a forest of trees creaking in the wind to the sounds of birds, frogs, and crickets, what does the music of the natural world say to you? Listen to the interactions between sounds, and pay attention to the conversations and dialogues.

Remember being a child and imitating the sounds of nature? Isolate one sound that you most resonate with. Trust your intuition and go with it. Start by joining that sound, perhaps humming playfully. Once you've joined, try making new sounds that harmonize, blending and extending the composition sound. Imagine the sound of nature as being part of a duet—together you are making harmony.

Build a Bridge

(Track 8)

A music-making experience with another person allows you to experience the feeling of being in harmony. Track 8 is a great example of an improvised dialogue between Tibetan and Native American flutes, a potent example of a soul-filled duet of cultures.

This practice moves beyond communication; it is communion. You can use nothing more than your voices or perhaps two instruments. It may be the same or different instruments. Create a dialogue by following the steps together: listen, unite, harmonize, and co-create.

Position yourself facing each other. The first step to harmonizing with others is always to listen. If you are both comfortable with eye contact and don't need to be looking at your instrument to play, it's powerful to keep an eye-to-eye connection. After all, the eyes are the seat of the soul.

Allow the first person to "speak" on the instrument or with his or her voice, but without using words. Respond naturally. Turn off your mind and body; activate your soul. Feel your souls connecting. Build upon the phrases. Contribute spontaneously to the wordless dialogue. See if you naturally access the shared muse that is guiding your collaboration. Feel the music come to a natural ending, a shared agreement of closing together. Visit youtube.com/ubdrumcircles and search for "Build a Bridge."

Create a Herd of Harmony

It is said that in certain African tribal villages, if a person is struggling, the community gathers around and chants that person's name until his or her soul is soothed and healed. The community encircles the person in sound, becoming a herd of harmony.

A modern variation is the group practice that my friend and sound healer Kristina Sophia of Musical Missions of Peace calls a "sound bubble." Have a person who needs soul healing stand in the center of the circle, with everyone gathered tightly around. Invite someone to start sounding the person's name. As everyone gradually joins in, you create a choir of angels invoking the healing energy of souls united. Feel the way each person's note amplifies the notes of others. Feel the sense of the soul's eternal transcendent nature.

You can also use this group practice to honor and show gratitude for someone. I once led a workshop in the giant sequoia forest at Far Horizons Retreat, where my group gathered around the cook to thank her by harmonizing her name on the final day of the retreat. The love and appreciation conveyed in sound brought tears to her eyes and allowed her to feel on a soul level our deep gratitude. It was our turn to feed her.

You can send harmony to any place it's needed by setting a group intention. Like a root tone, the intention is the key to the chord. Chant the name of the place in the world and become a prayer of peace and harmony in sound.

Play Your Part

(Track 9)

Feed your soul by joining a drum ensemble at a drum circle or by playing along with a traditional world rhythm from *The Healing Drum Kit*. To learn more world rhythms, seven rhythms from around the world are provided in the kit for ensemble playing.

One of the most popular rhythms is samba, which comes from Brazil. Samba is a parade rhythm played by thousands of percussionists in the streets of Bahia and Rio de Janeiro during Carnival. The instrumentation of the samba ensemble includes bells, shakers, *surdos* (bass drums), *pandeiros* (tambourine-style drums), *tamborim* (small frame drums), and *repenique* (snare drums). From the simplest job of playing the shakers to the more complex gig of the snare drum, each part is unique, yet they all line up. Listen to the parts of the play-along. For an example of the samba rhythm, visit youtube.com/ubdrumcircles.

ANNOTATED PLAYLIST FOR HARMONY

To stream this music, visit SoundsTrue.com/MusicMedicine.

1. "Return," Deirdre Ní Chinnéide, *Celtic Passage*
In the rich tradition of Celtic music, the bagpipes and tin whistle are harmonized with strings and keyboards. Notice how the different instruments interact, play together, move, and harmonize.

2. "Coro Coro," Geoff Johns, *Bakongo!*
In the spirit of the Orisha tradition, this beautiful expression of harmony calls to the spirits, often represented by nature's elements. Hear the rich harmonies of women's voices singing together, and let your soul be moved by the spiritual devotion and reverence spoken through harmony.

3. "Chola's Groove," Pepe Danza, *Drum Prayers*
A driving rhythm creates a palette of harmony between flute and saxophone, chasing each other around in improvised solos and coming together in this composition. Notice the interplay of drum and saxophone, and the dialogue and conversation of music's medicine in harmony.

4. "Mbira Kosamdela," Shaman's Dream, *African Dream*
The music of the Zimbabwean thumb piano, the *mbira*, calls us into harmony with sounds of nature. In the Lingala language of Democratic

Republic of the Congo, *kosamdela* means "we pray." This prayer is sung by Dido Tshibangu and accompanied by seed shakers, gourd, clay drums, and nature's symphony of birds and waters.

5. "Aum—Sri Ma," Chloë Goodchild, *Thousand Ways of Light*
Chant along with Chloë Goodchild, founder of The Naked Voice (thenakedvoice.com), a training program for the use of voice in sound healing and spiritual awakening. Let your soul be enveloped by the gradually building harmonies. Join the choir of angels chanting to "MA," the Great Mother, with soul-filled devotion.

6. "A Wish," Hamza El Din, *A Wish*
The beautiful music of the *oud,* an ancient lute, weaves together with an ensemble of guitar, voice, piano, and frame drum in traditional Nubian music preserved by Hamza El Din, despite the loss of his homeland due to its water crisis.

7. "Berceuse [Drum Negrito]," Ricardo Cobo, *Guitar Lullaby*
Colombian guitarist Richard Cobo soothes our soul with a gorgeous lullaby in harmonies that soften the melody line and call us to peace.

8. "Meditation," Nawang Khechog, *Music as Medicine*
This recording reestablishes the inner harmony of the soul, a meditation that layers a tapestry of keyboard chords with both Tibetan and Native American flutes.

9. "Samba Rhythm," Christine Stevens, *The Healing Drum Kit*
Listen and play along in an experience of ensemble medicine that uses the many different percussion elements of the Afro-Brazilian rhythm samba. Can you hear each different percussion instrument and how they all come together in this traditional rhythm ensemble?

6

Silence: Medicine for the Mind

Hello darkness, my old friend
I've come to talk with you again
Within the sound of silence

—PAUL SIMON AND ART GARFUNKEL, "THE SOUND OF SILENCE"

I t is said that before any sound, there is silence. Within silence, there is power. My experience in Iraq showed me how sonic expression leads to deep silence, and how that silence is a tool for peace.

By the second day of our training program in Iraq, the drum circles were beginning to gel. I was worried, though, because later that day I had to give a lecture on the science of drumming through our Kurdish and Arabic translators. I'd never spoken in front of a multilanguage group, and I can tell you that the experience was frustrating and slow. I spoke one sentence, and then waited for both translators to speak before I could go on to the next sentence.

Finally, after an hour of trenching through the mud of language, I suddenly realized the impending three-ring circus of the question-and-answer session. Spontaneously, I suggested we divide into separate language groups for the Q&A. While the translators informed the group of my suggestion, I waited . . . and waited.

No one moved. There was nothing but the sound of people whispering to each other, like bees swarming a hive. I asked what was going on, and the translators explained in five words that I'll never forget: "They don't want to separate."

This marked a turning point in our training. We had reached a level of cohesion that overruled the practical idea of splitting up. I nodded my head in agreement and stood by my flip chart, ready for the first question. Instead, a young Kurdish man picked up his flute and began to play a melody. An Arab man immediately joined him on his drum.

The next thing I knew, the whole room had erupted. My flip chart was pushed out of the way as participants played instruments and formed a dance line. A band of Kurds and Arabs, Sunni and Shia, emerged to accompany the dance. I was pulled into the chain, hooking arms and rocking back and forth, led by a man whirling prayer beads in the air.

After more than an hour of the spontaneous weaving of Kurdish and Arabic rhythms and dance, the music began to quiet down. As we returned to our seats, I wasn't the only one with an expression of surprised joy on my face.

The group spontaneously fell into stillness, sitting together in peace. It was not the uncomfortable feeling we had had at the start of our program, when language barriers had prevented the possibility of dialogue. This was the silence that sings of satisfaction and accomplishment. And in the silence, I could still hear the powerful rhythms beating, the songs playing, and the harmonies of cultures dancing together, made audible in the silence, like light shining in darkness.

From Sound to Silence

According to noted sound healing expert Jill Purce, "The purpose of sound is silence."[1] Common expressions show how important the music of silence is for peace of mind. We say that silence is golden. We associate peace and quiet. We recognize the incubating ideas hidden in a moment of silence as a pregnant pause. We say, "Words are valuable, but silence is more precious." We honor the passing of a loved one with a moment of silence.

Silence is defined as the absence of sound. Yet it turns out that absolute silence is nearly impossible. Decibels measure sound, yet zero decibels can only be created in an anechoic chamber, or a sensory-deprivation booth. Here, the record length of time a human can endure total silence is less than an hour, around forty-five minutes. While inside the chamber, two distinct sounds arise: a high pitch and a low pitch, not from outside but from the inside—it is the human biology singing. Scientists suggest that the high pitch is the sound of our neurology, and the low pitch is the sound of our blood circulating. The hum of our bodies cannot be silenced.

We also face the challenge of mental noise in daily life. The mind gets cluttered, chatting incessantly about the past or future, worries and doubts. Its song is cacophonous. External sound also affects our internal mental symphony. That is why churches and temples are filled with the music of silence, just as libraries create spaces of concentration and focus. There's no doubt that our sonic environment affects our minds. We would probably all agree intuitively that meditation is more challenging in a noisy sound environment. Inner silence is the soundscape of meditation.

Noise Pollution

Noise is on the rise. Today, thirty million Americans suffer from environment-related deafness.[2] Roughly twenty-five million Americans have tinnitus, a condition of ringing in the ears, and 15 percent of Americans have high-frequency hearing loss due to loud sounds or noise in work or in life.[3] In his book *Zero Decibels,* George Michelson Foy measured the soundscape of urban life; he recorded New York City subway trains at 94 to 98 decibels, which is 100 percent over the Occupational Safety and Health Administration standards for workplace noise exposure.[4]

Since 1980, the World Health Organization has been concerned about the growing amount of traffic noise and occupational noise pollution, documenting the toll it takes on our mental and physical health. A study from Stockholm's Institute of Environmental Medicine showed that noise pollution resulted in an increase in health problems, including hearing impairment, sleep disturbance, and psychological agitation. Noise levels of 80 decibels and greater increased aggression and actually decreased helping behaviors. The study found that more than 30 percent of Europeans are exposed to sound levels exceeding 55 decibels at night, a level of noise that is disturbing to sleep.[5] In *Healing at the Speed of Sound,* authors Don Campbell and Alex Doman offer a comprehensive review of sound and noise pollution, with helpful practices for protecting our hearing.[6] For more information, see healingatthespeedofsound.com.

Noise pollution can exist inside our minds as well. From mindfulness classes in hospitals to workplace wellness programs, learning to quiet the mind is ever-more important. A survey found that more than twenty million Americans—about one out of eleven—had meditated in the previous year.[7] A growing number of medical centers offer meditation classes to patients for stress reduction, wellness, and symptom management.

Take a moment to ask yourself where you need the sound of silence in your life. How do you quiet your mind? Do you have favorite music that helps take you into silence? Is your life filled up, with no space?

The Art of Silence

Silence gives music space to breathe and gives listeners time to digest. Without spaces, music would be out of breath, exhausted, and unbalanced. Sound familiar? The musical notation for silence is literally called a rest, reminding us that music needs its moments of repose as much as we do. Rests count in musical notation, and musicians count rests when playing music. Especially for the rhythm players, silence beats on. It's what you leave out that creates the space that makes a rhythm.

You may have noticed that music designed for relaxation contains more space, both in the melody and rhythm. Long notes call our ears to listen for the sweet moment when the sound fades away. Time slows down and elongates itself like a slow exhale. Instead of pulsing beat, time fluctuates and changes, which is called *rubato,* meaning "stolen time." A slow rhythm helps calm our bodies, while the absence of tempo frees the mind. That is why our minds find peace in the sound of wind chimes or the sustained tone of a singing bowl. We hear these sounds in nature—the way the sound of falling raindrops sprinkles a rooftop or the rise and fall of wind whispering across an open field of dry grass.

A sign of mastery in musicians and composers is the use of silence. You hear it in the tasty playing of space by trumpet player Miles Davis in cool jazz. He balances his artistry between play and pause, rhythm and repose. The meditative flute melodies of Native America or Tibet also reflect this style, playing more silence than notes. *(Listen to tracks 2, 6, and 7 in the online silence playlist.)*

Silence as a musical element pushes music to new realms. Known for his radical use of silence, avant-garde composer John Cage wrote 4'33" ("Four minutes and thirty-three seconds") in 1952. In this composition, the performer or performers sit on stage in complete silence for the specified time. Even though the musicians do not play, sounds do happen in the audience. Cage's composition called both performer and audience to hear silence as an equally important element of music, and reversed roles. The audience became part of the composition.

Four Types of Musical Silence

Silence exists before, during, and after music. Yet, even before the music, there is an original silence that is the source of musical expression.

1. *Original Silence*. Silence is the cocoon of artistry. Gestation often happens in silence, where deep seeds of our individual artistic expression are found. There is no standard incubation time in creativity. Each silent idea, song, rhythm, or vision has its own rhythm. Even when we are silent, creative work is happening. This source silence is mysterious.

It is evident in the curious compositional genius that Ludwig van Beethoven heard through his deaf ears. Original silence calls mystics to the desert and seekers to silent retreats. In the true sense of paradox, sound is born in silence.

Paul McCartney tells the story of how he wrote the modern classic "Yesterday." He woke up humming the melody, coming directly out of the silence of dream time. In his acceptance speech at the White House for the Gershwin Prize for Popular Song, McCartney said, "I don't know where the music comes from; I'm just glad it comes."[8] Perhaps he tapped into the source that can only be described as a silent vibration, birthing itself through artists into song.

You can cultivate silence in your life, like tending to seedlings of plants. You can learn to recognize its power as a force of creativity, a hidden soil rich with possibility. In the quiet mind, you will cultivate seeds of creative inspiration that lie within you.

2. *Silence before Music*. Silence before music calls the listener to attention and calls performers to their hearts. Before the music starts, especially in a group experience, a choir of silence precedes the first sound. If the conductor just went directly to the podium and immediately started waving the baton, there'd never be music, just cacophony. When the conductor lifts the baton, the orchestra begins in the pause of preparation.

Notice the moments that precede sound or motion in the music of your life. Perhaps it's taking a moment to be centered before entering a meeting or paying attention to the breath that precedes spoken word. Feel the silence and its rich preparation to fully support your next sound.

3. *Silence within Music.* According to Benedictine monk Brother David Steindl-Rast, "It's the silence between the notes that gives them meaning and grace."[9] Silence within music can be heard in all the other elements. Silence within rhythm creates pause and punctuation. We feel it in a space before and after a strong accented beat or in the upbeat syncopation that is just off the regular pulse. It surprises us. Silence within melody creates phrasing and lyrical lines. The silence that sets up a long note at the end of a song causes audiences to cheer when it finally ends. Silence within harmony is heard in dialogue between voices, the silence between phrases that creates the turn-taking of call and response.

Similarly, a pause between the words in the music of language is one of the most powerful tools used by public speakers. The pause inserted within the speech is what draws the attention and emphasis to whatever comes next.

Notice how often people pause within their speech. Notice the moments of pause within your own sentences. Go into the pregnant pause. What does it birth in you? How does your pause help a listener hear the deeper meaning of your words?

4. *Silence after Music.* There is a shimmering quality that follows the last note of a musical performance. In the immediate quiet, we feel the vibration of the music running through us. Whether we are the listener or the music maker, the silence allows musical digestion and absorption. Sometimes we even feel a rush come over us that, ironically, is stronger than the music itself. As John Cage said, "Silence allows the listener's music to be heard."[10] The silence after music calls us to ourselves. Great musical movement creates sonic stillness. In the absence, we feel the presence.

In drum circles, the powerful silence after the last beat is often the moment of the greatest awareness of group success. It's ironic that the moment that creates the greatest sense of togetherness and connectedness is often the space more than the sound. Silence after music is also a hallmark of mantra meditation practices, where chanting gets progressively quieter, becoming more inward, until it fades into silence.

Notice whether you leave space after the songs in your life. Do you rush into the next experience, or do you take time to digest life's music? Have you ever felt the richness of lingering in a beautiful experience, the resonance that travels deeper into your mind, body, and soul? What would it feel like to have more space after each song, each movement, each significant symphony in your life?

The Creative Mind

In this ongoing theme of what music *does* for us, as well as what it *undoes*, when you deactivate the thinking mind, you discover a greater voice: the creative mind. Its song is activated in silence; it is a genius of creativity that is nurtured in quiet. If you've ever had a great idea just after you've been sitting in silence or right when you wake up in the morning, then you are familiar with this principle of the creative mind.

This is why I play music early in the morning, before my mind can wake up. It is a race of consciousness. If I don't play music first thing, my mind beats me and begins to play its cacophony of tasks, worries, and busy thoughts. I prefer the music of silence, as well as the wisdom and creativity I've come to know in its playing.

Resting—The Principle of Silence

In music and in life, silence is called a "rest." Every living thing must rest. We balance speaking and listening, doing and being, moving and pausing. On the seventh day, God rested. So why is it hard to give ourselves a day of rest? As children, we enjoy naptime in kindergarten. Yet somehow, unless we live in the siesta culture of Latin America or practice Shabbat, the Jewish tradition of a day of rest, we don't get enough rest to maintain the health that helps our bodies and minds sing like a well-tuned instrument. We can forget the importance of rest for our lives the same way we can forget that silence is part of music.

When I created *The Healing Drum Kit,* I included the controversial rhythm of resting. To play this rhythm, you simply place your hands on the drum and do nothing. It was my version of John Cage. The play-along soundtrack has spacious piano music that is rubato; in other words, it is played in free time.

Before the kit was published, I tested the rhythm of resting on a few people, including my sister-in-law, who was raising three children all under the age of eight. I watched her whole body relax and her breathing deepen as she first experienced the rhythm of resting. She nearly burst into tears because she was so starved of time in which to be still. I realized the importance of just being with an instrument without needing to play it, to just make a connection. I also saw how quickly sound affects someone who is open to receive it. In just three minutes, her mind, body, and spirit had transformed.

The Shadow Side of Silence

Silence is not always golden. It can be dark and restrictive, terrifying and forceful, mysterious and empty. Silence is associated with death. When sound lingers into silence, we call it "dying off." Silence holds a negative connotation related to trauma and disempowerment—causing the silencing of an individual's voice. Keeping secrets is a necessary coping strategy, yet it's the withholding, the silencing, that causes psychological and physiological problems.

Silence is often uncomfortable. We fill our homes with sound, becoming conditioned to living in an active sonic environment of television and radio. No wonder the record in a sound deprivation chamber was only forty-five minutes. Silence can be scary: it can cause a sense of urgency, and we rush to fill the space. We do what it takes to avoid the void.

Musical instruments remind us that we have to be empty in order to make sound. The empty hole in the guitar under the strings of the body is called the sound hole, the place that allows the voice of the guitar to be heard. Likewise, the Tibetan singing bowl must be empty to resonate. We are like instruments: our empty places may be sound holes that are making space for our greater voice to come through and to receive inspiration and creativity. As we embrace silence, we hear its songs.

The Science of Silence

If you've ever wondered what effect silence can have on mind and body, Luciano Bernardi, MD, from the University of Pavia, Italy, has come up with some answers. A rock guitarist in his youth and a Renaissance guitarist today, Bernardi wanted to know which elements of music—rhythm, melody, or silence—were most effective in calming the mind and body. Subject s listened to six different musical selections: slow, medium, and fast classical music, techno, rap, and soothing raga music from India. To test silence, a two-minute pause was randomly inserted between the music tracks on two occasions. The random pauses allowed researchers to avoid giving subjects a sense of predictability, which could create a conditioning effect. The research team measured standard markers of relaxation: breathing rate, pulmonary blood flow, blood pressure, and heart rate.[11]

Results of Bernardi's study initially went as expected. Rhythm showed a significant impact, with fast tempos increasing breathing and heart rate, while slower music reduced them. But the surprising result came during the random periods of silence between the music selections. It was during the silence rather than during the sound that the greatest evidence of relaxation occurred: decreased blood pressure, slower ventilation rate, and lowered heart rate. In fact, silence outperformed all other music conditions.

This study has great implications for how we can access the medicine of silence. Like the practice of tension and release used in progressive muscle relaxation, music has its own pattern of presence and absence that creates relaxation, a tandem effect of sound and silence. We can apply the results of this science by selecting slower tempos to entrain our biology in the direction of peace and calm or by choosing faster tempos to excite our natural rhythm. By allowing some silence between songs, we can access greater levels of relaxation and quieting of our minds. And we can enter the silence that follows the music to discover our inner sense of tranquility and relaxation.

The Silent Prescription

You may have heard of an interesting phenomenon that demonstrates the power of the mind known as the placebo effect. When given a placebo, such as a "dummy" pill, 35 to 59 percent of people showed positive results, as if they had taken the actual medicine.[12] Based upon a Harvard study from Beth Israel Deaconess Medical Center, researchers who tested a placebo for patients with irritable bowel syndrome (IBS) found that in 59 percent of cases, subjects demonstrated adequate relief from symptoms after taking the placebo.[13] In other words, our minds can change our biology. Likewise, your belief in music makes it a powerful force of healing in your life. Your belief in yourself makes you a powerful force as well.

Quieting the Mind

Researchers have discovered some interesting on-and-off switches in the brain when it is engaged in meditation. A group at Aarhus University Hospital in Denmark used brain scans—functional magnetic resonance imaging (fMRI)—to test Zen meditators, all of whom had at least eight years' experience meditating. The subjects were asked to switch between forty-five-second periods of meditation and random thinking, while researchers took images of the subjects' brains in real time.

The results showed that a neural switch does occur when meditating, with two very different brain patterns emerging. Meditation created activation in the prefrontal cortex and the basal ganglia, which are the areas of the brain involved in sharpened focus, attention, insights, and deep emotions.[14] Specifically, the basal ganglia, which function in precise, controlled movements (like Zen archery), became more active. Simultaneously, deactivation occurred in two larger brain areas—the occipital gyrus and the anterior cingulate cortex—which are responsible for visual orientation, conscious activity, and willful action. The overall result showed a quiet mind that turned off larger brain areas and concerns about time or place, with a simultaneous increase in a small brain area leading to focus, relaxation, and positive emotions. Again, it's what silence *undoes* that makes it medicine for the mind.

Similar results were seen in a study by pioneering stress researcher Herbert Benson, MD, at Harvard Medical School. Using the same fMRI brain imaging, researchers tested kundalini meditators with four years of experience, looking at how repeated meditation affects the mind. Subjects performed two twelve-minute meditations with a thinking exercise in between. All subjects meditated by silently repeating a calming phrase—a mantra—while also focusing on breathing.

Again, researchers found prefrontal cortex activation during meditation, as well as a specific activation of an area of the brain involved in empathy and emotion—that is, the cingulate cortex. Simultaneously, most of the brain became inactive, silenced by the meditation practice.[15] The second meditation, after the thinking exercise, showed an even greater effect, demonstrating that repeated practice does strengthen mindfulness.

The silence of inner words or song when using a mantra or counting breaths turns out to be significant in achieving a quiet mind. A team of researchers at the University Hospital in Lund, Sweden, found that counting out loud creates a mental picture different from that achieved by silent internal speech. By testing meditators who counted their breath either out loud or silently, researchers found that external speech activated auditory and motor areas that can distract from meditation, while internal speech activated prefrontal areas that are part of focusing attention. It's the silence that makes the neurological shift.[16]

Minding the Silence

Research shows that quieting the mind takes practice, training, and guidance. Jon Kabat-Zinn at the University of Massachusetts Medical School developed a training program called mindfulness-based stress reduction (MBSR), which bridges science and spirit, creating a protocol that could be standardized in research and practiced in medical centers. With numerous studies published to date, the MBSR approach has gained a great deal of scientific acceptance and is applied worldwide. In the eight-week training program, participants learn such skills as mindful breathing, body-scan meditation, mindful walking, loving-kindness, and rest. Silence is a featured component, with a seven-hour silent retreat during the sixth week of training.[17]

Researchers who used MBSR in an experiment with employees in the workplace found an improved immune function, more frontal brain activation, and reduced burnout in the employees who took the course. An additional important finding came four months later, when subjects were retested and still demonstrated positive results as compared with those without the training. Regular meditation, along with a seven-hour immersion in silence about every two months, is a prescription for a quiet mind, stronger health, and a more positive experience in the workplace.[18]

In summary, silence comes to mind by deactivating larger brain areas, including any concerns about where we are or what we are thinking about, and by turning on a heightened, focused attention. Thoughts can be tuned out and turned down, like adjusting switches on a soundboard at a concert, so that one channel remains—the soloist is the prefrontal cortex, facilitating our focus, attention, insights, and deep emotions. Our brains are amazingly adaptable, what science calls *neural plasticity*. Our neurology continues to change, and positive effects continue to become amplified with practice that incorporates silence. It pays to invest in learning an evidence-based, spiritually grounded meditation practice to bring the benefits of silence into our minds.

The Spirit of Silence

From Quaker meetings to Benedictine monastic life, the spirituality of silence creates the resonance of contemplation, depth, and direct communion with the Creator. The Psalms say, "Be still and know that I am God." Christian mystics practice contemplative or centering prayer, which has grown out of the seventh-century philosophy of Quietism, using silence as a bridge to direct communion with God. Hindu guru and musician Sri Chinmoy said, "Silence is the source of everything. It is the source of music, and it is music itself."[19] Paramahansa Yogananda sang to God in his chant "I Give You My Soul Call": "Come out of the silent song; come out of your cave of silence."[20] Even Gandhi devoted one day a week to total silence, a practice he held to with great integrity, no matter what dignitary came to visit.

The Lakota sacred teachings say that the Great Mystery moved into motion the polarity of silence and sound. Before sound, there was the great void. From the silence came the sound, and from the sound came the substance of the universe. In the Lakota language, the word for this original silence is *skan skan wakan*. The Lakota word *skan* translates as "move"; thus, *skan skan* literally translates as "move move," which, through Lakota understanding, is "moving movement" or making something happen. It is this generative silence from which all sound, all movement, and all creation are born—an original silence.

In the Lakota tradition, seekers go on a vision quest—or *hanbleceya*, which translates as "crying for a vision"—spending four days and nights without food or water in silence in nature's sanctuary. It's a practice of vacancy, emptying, and deep listening that happens when your ears begin to hear the music of nature and the voice of inner guidance.

Buddha's Ears

Buddhism has a long and profound tradition of silence. The Buddha plays no instrument, but if silence is a sound, Buddha is a maestro. Statues and artwork depict the Buddha with closed mouth and long, prominent ears, quietly listening in peace. The story goes that after years of attempts at enlightenment, Buddha sat in silent meditation for forty-nine days under the bodhi tree until he became "awake." It was silence, not sound, that woke him up.

Darkness, My Old Friend

In *The Music of Silence,* Brother Steindl-Rast spoke to the music of silence found in the darkness of night and honored by silent Benedictine monks, whose chanting is the only sound that breaks the stillness. He explains that in the monastic tradition, nighttime is called Compline, which means "completion." Like the silence at the end of the music, Compline completes the day. It is a time of rest and repose, reflection and integration. The dark of night becomes the dark of predawn, as the next canonical hour that follows is Vigil—the night watch, the womb of silence. It is in the silence of early premorning that many monastic traditions awaken to commune with the spirit of God found in silence.

Brother Steindl-Rast referred to the time between Compline and Vigil—between nightfall and predawn—as "the hole between the threads of days."[21] This reminds me of the story among the famous Native blanket weavers of Chimayó, New Mexico, who say that a hole in the weaving is not a mistake; rather, it's the space where Spirit enters. The hole is where the holy comes through. The same applies in the acoustic tapestry of our lives. In our awareness of silence and the presence in the absence, we create an inner monastery for Spirit to enter.

The Mind's Ear

If mystics see the light in darkness, perhaps they also hear the song in silence? Spiritual teachers of traditions ranging from Christian to Hindu talk about the mind's eye or the third eye, a single point of spiritual focus that is filled with the light of Divine presence. But what about the mind's other senses? Are we so visually oriented that we've forgotten that Spirit speaks in sound?

Imagine the mind's ear, a single point of sonic focus that can hear the inaudible, tune into Divine silence, and attune to the vibration of *ohm,* the holy spirit, the sweet vibrational hum of the universe. There is an ear training that occurs as we uplift ourselves and raise our inner vibration. We hear differently, detecting music in the sounds in nature or even in surprising places in normal life. A spiritually tuned individual begins to hear the beauty of life more than the noise, the voice of guidance born in stillness, and the song in the silence.

Instruments of Silence

We all have within us an instrument of silence: our breath. Long recognized as a tool for quieting the mind, the breath is the ultimate human expression of the element of air; it is the breeze that blows our thoughts away and fills our lungs. As we breathe consciously, we listen to our own inner sound and we quiet our mind.

There are also instruments that come from a sacred lineage that can carry us to silence. Strings of bells often hang outside temples in Asia, played randomly by the wind's breath, like wind chimes on a porch.

Singing bowls from the Tibetan sound-healing tradition create long, sustained tones, which help us listen for the tapering off into silence. These instruments have been used for thousands of years, dating back to pre-Buddhist Bön culture, which used singing bowls to create a hypnotic state of consciousness. As such, the bowls were said to have been played by lamas who were initiated in the use of sound. To this day, we often hear a bell call us to quiet in schools, temples, and meditation groups.

The Medicine of Silence—Resting Medicine

Sometimes we teach what we need to learn. Through a serious injury of my own, I learned the potency of the medicine of resting for a crucial part of any musician's body: the ears.

As a drum-circle leader, my years of loud sound exposure caught up with me, and I was diagnosed with tinnitus, a ringing in my ears. At its initial onset, it was painful. The pressure in my ears kept building, and I constantly needed to pop my jaw to relieve the tension. There is no known treatment for this condition except reduced exposure to loud sound. The condition threw me into a state of confusion, as I considered that my career in drumming was over.

After weeks of depression, I decided to try an innovative approach. I headed to Joshua Tree, California, for some deep quiet. The desert's silence was my music medicine. Sitting outside, under a thatched palapa in the quiet desert soundscape, I began to feel my ears open up again. After three days immersed in sacred quietude, I began to feel a sense of hope. The ringing did not go away, but the pain did.

Because we can't close our ears like we can close our eyes, it takes strong measures to create the healing silence of the desert in an urban environment. I took time every day to give my ears a rest by wearing earplugs and noise-canceling headphones. Eventually, I recovered. Much more carefully and with heightened awareness of the volume, I am now able to work in drum circles again by using musician's earplugs to protect the ears I recovered through resting.

Resting the Mind

The brain in silence is naptime for the mind. Otherwise we're always thinking, even in our sleep. The problem with resting the mind is that there is no on/off switch. Thinking is not the same as resting the body. In fact, sometimes moving the body helps quiet the mind. Mindful walking, jogging, dancing, yoga, or even a good workout can be "active meditation."

Playing music can be another form of active meditation, as can playing drums, improvising, or chanting. When you play music, you become present. If you think about it too much, especially when drumming, you screw up. But when you combine drumming and silence, you create a rich opportunity to unmind your mind and achieve rest. Whether you get there by stillness or movement, the mind needs rest, a break from the cacophony of thought.

Resting the Body

Sleep deprivation affects many people. More than half of American adults say they experience a sleep problem almost every night, and sixty-three percent say their weekly sleep needs are not being met.[22] Studies show an increased mortality risk for those getting fewer than six or seven hours of sleep per night.[23] No matter how much rest you get, high stress can cause a feeling of restlessness. It's the quality of sleep that is so important to our restoration and renewal—and that is the medicine of resting.

Final Chorus

Silence is an element of music that occurs before, during, and after music. Through the gateway of silence, we touch the original silence that births creative inspiration and offers rich communion with the Divine. The benefits of silence for the mind extend into health, healing, spirituality, and restoration. The medicine of silence helps us tune out the mental chatter and become more aware of why we cultivate silence; it helps us rest, digest, and gestate our higher creative calling. For the mind, the music of silence leads to peace and greater creativity.

GUIDED PRACTICES FOR THE
MEDICINE OF SILENCE

These practices will support you in tuning in to the medicine of silence and incorporating the principle of resting into your life. Take a moment to ask yourself where you need the sound of silence in your life. When and where could you use more peace and quiet? What stops you from getting the rest you need?

The first set of practices gives you ways to invoke and receive silence, including a conscious listening practice with a recommended playlist of music specifically created to quiet the mind. The second set of practices shows how to express the music of silence, both alone and with others. As always, follow what resonates with you and bring the healing benefits of silence into the music of your life.

Guided Practices for Conscious Listening

Questing for Quiet

(Track 10 from the online silence playlist)

Begin noticing both the noise and the silence in the external environments of your daily life. Notice that your mind has ears, and see how your thoughts and feelings are sensitive to sound environments.

Move through a day with the curiosity of where you can find quiet. Take a tour of your home, workplace, or somewhere in nature, and find places and spaces where quiet exists. If you have wind chimes, sit and listen to the silence between the notes and to the wind playing its song. Notice how the quiet changes your breath. As you breathe, make a sound like a sigh on the out-breath, then listen as the sound fades—you have become your own singing bowl. Enter the silence.

If you can't go directly to a place in nature, take a moment to imagine a scene of peace and quiet, a serene setting. Play track 10 from the silence playlist on page 128 and hear the sounds of the rainforest. Picture yourself in a beautiful, open grove within the tropical rainforest or in a great, expansive desert with a quiet wind gently blowing against tiny grains of sand. You may prefer to envision being outside after a snowfall or the quiet of being inside a cave by a toasty fire, hearing the crackles light the soundscape of quietude. Wherever you prefer to be in nature's musical silence, let your mind rest and enjoy a moment of peace of mind.

Pay attention and embrace the sound of silence in the darkness of night. This is the canonical hour of Compline. Feel the rhythm of settling into sleep, the rest that follows the busy activities of the day. Make a conscious switch into the rhythm of rest. If you are an early riser, notice the silence of darkness that comes in the predawn, the canonical hour of Vigil, and live in a rhythm of awareness of the spiritual meaning of darkness, the entry point to Spirit that awaits in quiet moments of the special hours of silence.

Listening to the Space between the Notes

(Tracks 1–8)

I've created a playlist of relaxing meditative music, chosen for having more space between the notes and a slow beat, or rubato, creating a peaceful state. You may also have favorite recordings of singing bowls, chant, flutes, nature, or other sources that give you a sense of rest or a quiet mind.

Begin with a few deep, even breaths, allowing your mind to be embraced by the gentle rhythm of your breath as it gradually, effortlessly begins to slow and deepen. Tuning in to your breath is its own soundtrack and your own instrument of silence; doing so can establish an immediate sense of peace. There is a rich moment of silence between the inhale and exhale of breath. Hold the silence before and after you breathe, and just be with your breath. As you exhale, empty your mind.

Invite the mind's ear to listen to the music in the silence playlist. Listening to the silence within music is like looking at art from the perspective of the negative space. We can look at either the lines and colors or the empty spaces. Let the music draw your attention into a single focus. Listen for moments of absence, where there are no notes or beats. Notice which silence feels best to you: before, during, or after the music?

When the piece concludes, pause for a moment of digestion. Notice how your breathing or heartbeat may have changed. Pause the music until you are ready to continue.

Sound Savasana

(All tracks)

Savasana is a Sanskrit term referring to a yoga pose, an *asana* of receiving and resting. You can use this position to amplify the effects of conscious listening and to bring the resting medicine into your mind and body. Lie down on your back in a comfortable position with your arms flat on the ground and palms up. Place your heels together, allowing your feet to fall out in any way that's comfortable. Set your intention to be completely open to music—listening not just with your ears, but with your whole body, mind, and spirit. Let the sound wash over you. Focus only on the task of listening. Allow your mind's ear to tune into the sounds. Notice how your body begins to breathe more deeply.

When each recording is complete, take a moment to be grateful to the composer and musicians. Rest in the quietude, the space between songs.

Sound Break

The challenge of silence is that we cannot close our ears like we can close our eyes. We have to use earplugs or headphones. I've noticed that life today is filled with more earbuds and headphones than ever. Airplanes are packed with passengers wearing noise-canceling headphones that can be plugged into a sound source or that simply bring silence to the ears of the listeners. Something happens to our other senses when the auditory is turned down. We often think better, feel a clearer mind, and find a way to breathe more deeply and relax.

Give your ears a restorative sound break by wearing earplugs or noise-canceling headphones for a period of time. Create a sound break, decreasing the decibel exposure and giving more silence to your mind. Notice when you could use more silence in your day and test it out. You may notice you can concentrate better immediately or that this practice provides a nice break from life's soundtrack. I have been using earplugs and noise-canceling headphones, even combining both at the same time, to reduce the pain of my tinnitus. The silence is music to my ears.

Try a full dosage of seven hours in a silent retreat, as was recommended in the medical mindfulness studies. Researchers found silent retreats to be useful about once every eight weeks. You may want to go to a quiet place in nature or just take a break from talking for a day. Conclude your time of silence with a gradual reentry into the sound of life. Notice how clear your mind becomes. Consciously carry the silence with you throughout the rest of the day.

Guided Practices for Expressing

Silent Song

(Track 5)

Probably one of the oldest practices of musical silence comes from the Eastern tradition of mantra chanting. This practice begins with external chanting and gradually moves to the internalizing of the song in the mind as the outer voice fades into silence. Because beauty holds our attention, this practice allows us to lose our mind in sound. The silence that follows is golden indeed.

As it is said in the Eastern philosophy of yoga, "As the breath, so flows the mind." Chant elongates the breath. The extension of this practice goes beyond singing and moves into an internal state of peace and calm when the chant concludes.

Take fifteen minutes to chant. It may be a mantra you know, a simple repeated phrase, or a prayer. Or you can join Deva Premal in chanting the *moola mantra* (track 5 in the silence playlist). Repetition is comforting and allows the body to slow down in deep breaths that support sounding the music and that also create a meditative state of mind. At the end of fifteen minutes, sit in silence for five minutes and notice the effect on your mind. Be with the quietude that follows the chant. Notice the silence that has come through the song.

Silent Drum

(Track 9)

In drumming, the rhythm becomes a mantra that captures our attention. The act of drumming can deactivate mental thought and activate primal trance. Drumming is a form of active meditation that helps if you find it challenging to sit still and be silent.

Create a sacred space where you can settle in. Prepare to drum by making sure you are holding your drum in a comfortable position. Take a few deep breaths. Place your hand or mallet on the drum and begin in gratitude. Play a simple pulse, rhythm, or whatever feels good to you. Don't think. You may drum to music, such as the "Relaxing Rhythms" track from *The Healing Drum Kit* (see track 9 in the silence playlist), or you can make up your own calming rhythm.

Drum for a minimum of four minutes and allow yourself to settle in. Continue drumming until you lose track of time. When you are ready, fade your drumming into silence. Put down your drum and focus on your breath. Feel the rhythm of your breath. Stay in this meditative state for as long as you desire.

Speaking in Silence

The sound of silence can be practiced in daily speech. Try creating more silence by waiting a beat before responding in conversations. Notice how the pause affects the connection between listener and speaker. How does it change the tonality of the dialogue? What music is born between you?

Have you ever noticed a moment of unspoken connection through silence, perhaps a moment when you were gazing at another person and felt a moment of agreement and understanding? Like harmony in music, there is a shared silence when two or more people are coming from a place of peace. The practice of being in peaceful silence together can transform uncomfortable silence into comfortable communion and telepathic conversations spoken in silence.

Together with a willing partner, spend five minutes in silence. This is a challenging and rewarding practice that often brings up deep emotions. You can do this with eyes open, making eye contact with your partner for more intimacy, or with eyes closed. You may choose to synchronize your breathing or just notice that it happens through entrainment, without effort. Release the need to fill the space with sound. Allow silence to be the sound of a bridge between you, enhancing openness and trust. Release the need to fill the space and allow the connection to deepen.

Bowls and Bells

(Track 6)

Explore the power of playing a singing bowl or bells to achieve a quiet mind. You can experience the Tibetan sound-healing tradition with the sustained sound of the singing bowl, which provides a single tone that helps you focus and quiet your mind. The best way to choose a singing bowl is to play several, because every bowl is unique. The bowl that is right for you could be the one that is playing the note that your being represents. That is the medicine of this practice. Your body will guide you to the sound that most settles your mind.

To resonate a singing bowl, you must first of all hold it correctly. For the bowl to resonate, hold it on the open palm of your nondominant hand, facing upward. Make a straight plate with your palm so the bowl can resonate. The bowl should only touch your palm at the base. Using a wooden striker, you can play the bowl in two ways. First, you can sound it with the large end of the mallet in a single tone by striking the side of the bowl. Enjoy the sound and listen as it fades away, drawing you into silence.

Second, by pressing the beater into the outer shape of the bowl in a circular motion, you can resonate overtones and sustain the sound. It is much like sounding a crystal wineglass with your finger. Slow the movement to the edge of silence, finding the point where the bowl begins to stop vibrating at the level of sound. Again, breathe in the tonality and notice how it draws your mind into quiet. For more instruction, visit youtube.com/ubdrumcircles and search for "singing bowl."

Once you've practiced playing the singing bowl as your own silent meditation, you may want to explore offering it to another person or a group as a tool of musical silence together.

ANNOTATED PLAYLIST FOR SILENCE

To stream this music, visit SoundsTrue.com/MusicMedicine.

1. "Adrift on the Sea of Tranquility," Riley Lee, *Shakuhachi Water Meditations*
This is an example of the beautiful, peaceful sound of the Japanese *shakuhachi*
meditation flute. Shakuhachi flutes are made of bamboo and were traditionally played by monks wearing baskets over their heads to remove the sense
of performance and to retain an inward focus. This recording is a solo flute
with great spaces in between the notes that allow your heart to open as your
mind drifts away.

2. "Walking into the Himalaya to Meditate," Nawang Khechog,
Tibetan Meditation Music
Imagine yourself on a peaceful walk in nature as you listen to the gentle
sound of bells in the wind accompanying Nawang Khechog, Tibetan
Buddhist devotee and Grammy-nominated musician, who plays the Tibetan
bamboo flute of his homeland.

3. "Shiva's Flute," Shaman's Dream, *Kerala Dream*
The bansuri flute from India plays over a gentle keyboard and sitar, creating a
soundscape rich with the invitation to fall into peace. Let the quietude carry
you into a gentle calm, breathing with the waves of sound that wash over you.

4. "Samadhi," Shaman's Dream, *Kerala Dream*
The sound of sitar, gongs, and keyboard pads accompanies the sound of a
stream, creating a palette of peacefulness and floating without a set rhythm.
The rubato rhythm allows the spaciousness of deep breath and rest.

5. "Moola Mantra (Part 1)," Deva Premal, *Into Light: The Meditation Music
of Deva Premal*
This Sanskrit mantra is said to bring peace of mind, invoking the living
God for freedom from sorrow and suffering. It is a prayer of liberation,
love, and compassion. The translation is: "Oh Divine force, Spirit of All
Creation, Highest personality, Divine presence, manifest in every living being.

Supreme Soul manifested as the Divine Mother and as the Divine Father. I bow in deepest reverence."

Om sat chit ananda parabrahama
Purushothama paramatma
Sri bhagavati sametha
Sri bhagavate namaha
Hari om tat sat

6. "Above the Clouds," Cynth, *Flute Medicine—World Within, Volume 3*
Know for her three-album series of flute medicine, Cynth builds and plays her own medicine flutes. Recorded live in San Francisco's Grace Cathedral, this recording features the sound of wind chimes, singing bowls, and bamboo flute. Enter the spacious pauses between notes and the deep resonance of the crystal singing bowls and windchimes played by Sam Jackson. For more information, visit flutemedicine.com.

7. "Wisdom and Compassion," Nawang Khechog, *Tibetan Meditation Music*
The gift of silence is wisdom. Here Tibetan bamboo flutist Nawang Khechog includes the graciousness of space between notes to calm your mind.

8. "Ocean of Sound, Part 3," Pepe Danza, *Ocean of Sound*
The gentle sounds of chimes, bowls, and pan flutes offer expansive breaths that match the music's gentle sound, like ocean waves rocking you to peace and calm.

9. "Relaxing Rhythms Play-along," Christine Stevens, *The Healing Drum Kit*
To quiet the mind sometimes takes an active practice. Drumming has been an ancient tool to get into the body and out of the mind. Join me in this play-along track that I created to help you relax into the rhythm and release your thoughts.

10. "Meditative Rainforest," Jeffrey Thompson, *Meditative Rainforest*
Let nature guide you. Immerse yourself in the serene sounds of the Sri Lankan rainforest. The sounds of nighttime call you into the darkness of silence. Insects, frogs, and water dripping from leaf to leaf create a peaceful stillness.

7

Inner Music: Medicine for the Spirit

Thanks for the joy that you've given me
I want you to know I believe in your song
Rhythm and rhyme and harmony
You help me along makin' me strong.

—MENTOR WILLIAMS, "DRIFT AWAY"

One of the moments that taught me the most about the power of inner music happened when I was working with a young child in a healing center for the wounds of war.

I was invited to lead a drum circle at the Children's Rehabilitation Center in Sulaimaniya, Iraq, sponsored by Kurdistan Save the Children. The Center treated children with conditions ranging from amputated legs to heart disease to learning disabilities. When we arrived to demonstrate the drum circle for music therapy, we found that the center lacked a large gathering space, so we improvised and passed out drums in the waiting room, which was filled with children and their families.

I noticed a young boy, who looked to be eight or nine years old, slumped over in a wheelchair. He was missing both legs and looked depressed. But when I handed him a drum, he brightened up immediately. He sat up straight and started playing a traditional Kurdish beat. He had a fantastic sense of rhythm, much to the surprise of his parents and the therapists. His eyes were sparkling, and the shift in his energy was amazing. I could feel his spirit expressed on the drum as I got closer and tried to follow his rhythm. Without words, just demonstrating on his drum, he showed me how to play the Kurdish beat; he was giving me a lesson.

Meanwhile, drums were being passed out to the other children and parents. Before I knew it, the waiting room, which had once been filled with depressed faces, was filled with smiles and a unified spirit. The drum circle grew as therapists came from other parts of the center. I started to play an improvised melody on a flute that I had purchased in Iraq. The boy whose rhythm had started the whole thing kept on going, smiling and checking in with me with a nod of his head. When it was time to finish our program, I cued the group, speaking the numbers in Kurdish: 3–2–1–Stop! As everyone applauded, I pointed to the boy in the wheelchair, who acknowledged the applause with a bow.

As we were packing up the drums, I went over to the boy, whose parents were standing beside him in awe. He just looked at me and hugged the drum tightly. I knew he wanted to keep it, and I certainly would have given it to him, but instead I had to explain, through the translator, that I didn't have enough drums to give to all the children. I vowed that we would bring back enough drums for the center someday. He reluctantly handed me the drum. I nodded to him with my hand on my heart. He did the same.

As I walked away, I was filled with emotion. Suddenly, I heard a rhythm, but it wasn't on a drum. The boy was tapping out a beat with a pencil on the side of the metal wheelchair, a statement that burst my heart open. He did not need the drum to make his rhythm: the music was in him, not in the drum.

We kept our promise, returning the following year with drums for the center and were pleased to find the music therapy program flourishing under the direction of Raz, one of our trained facilitators and a physical therapist.

Make Me an Instrument

You are an instrument. You have a pitch, a timbre, a vibration, and a style. You are one of the seven billion unique instruments in the orchestra of humanity, playing the music each of us is here to play.

We hear the connection between our human instrument and musical instruments in phrases like "wound too tight" or "high-strung." We seek to find the right tuning of our inner strings without sounding or being too tight—or "uptight." We need to reduce the tension, literally, to stay in tune.

Playing an instrument is a practice of skill; becoming an instrument is a practice of consciousness. A well-known prayer attributed to Saint Francis of Assisi begins, "Make me an instrument of Your peace; Where there is hatred, let me sow love; Where there is discord, let me sow harmony ...Where there is doubt, let me sow faith. Where there is despair, let me sow hope. Where there is darkness, let me sow light."[1] And it goes on. This prayer expresses a desire that our resonance will retune doubt, despair, and darkness to the tone of harmony, hope, and light.

As you become aware of being an instrument, you make a paradigm shift from loving music to living music. Each moment of life deserves the fullest of who you are. There is a resounding state of wholeness derived by living the music of your spirit. Creativity is endless, vast as the horizon line on the ocean. As we grow as creative beings, our sound and rhythm develop, as do our silence and harmony, and we unfold into being the music of our unique true selves. In the words of Oscar Wilde, "You have set yourself to music. Your days are your sonnets. Life has been your art."[2]

In the circle of music medicine, you are the fifth element of music, the quintessence, which comes from the term *quint,* meaning "five." This essence is why you resonate with a particular instrument, song, or style of music. It is what generates the composition of musical expression that is your unique voice of creativity. It is the inner music at the core of your being. As human instruments, we are the music. The sixth-century Roman philosopher Boethius had a term for the music within us all: *musica humana.* When we are in harmony in body and soul, we are well-tuned instruments, singing our unique song in the symphony of life.

Musical Spirit

Once I was performing at a Unity church, and during the children's sermon, the minister asked the kids, "Where does music come from?" Two hands went up. The first child said, "The radio." The second child said, "From God." I called out from the audience and said, "From our heart."

What do you think? Does music come from the external, the eternal, or the internal?

There is internal music within every person. I call it our "musical spirit," a unique *esprit de corps* that lives at the core of our being. Musical spirit is an innate gift that needs to be cultivated and freed. Your musical spirit exists regardless of musical skill; it can be forgotten but never lost.

I once worked with an autistic child who was socially withdrawn, nonverbal, and highly agitated. He sat on the floor in the corner of the room, rocking back and forth. When I started to play a drumbeat on the conga, he would stand up and go to a drum I had placed near him in the room. At first he would copy my beat until he gradually started playing his own rhythms, and I became the one following him. It made me realize that musical spirit does not depend on skill or reading music; it's not inhibited by mental, emotional, or physical conditions. I've seen stroke patients with paralysis in their arms have bells strapped on their feet so they could tap their rhythm in a drum circle. It seemed nothing could stop their musical spirit.

Hopefully it doesn't take an injury or challenging health condition for you to recognize your inner musical spirit. Even trained musicians can become disconnected from their musical spirit, losing their connection to the joy that making music brings. Without spirit, their music may be technically impressive, but it lacks the energy of the artist. I am more moved by the beat played by a child whose inner music broke free and whose essence—which could not find words—began to speak than I am by the greatest technical performance that lacks spirit. Musical skill can enhance our expression, but musical spirit is essential.

As we express ourselves creatively, we bring forth the inner music that only we can play. It cannot be taught, because it is as natural as your heartbeat and as intimate as your breath. It's why music resonates with us so deeply. It's why all cultures have music. As Mickey Hart says, "No culture has existed without music . . . Music makes us human."[3]

Spirit Starved

Although it may be hard to measure in formal statistics, a growing trend in emotional and medical symptoms seems to point to an underlying loss of spirit. Author and visionary Jonathan Ellerby, PhD, coined the term "inspiration deficit disorder," which he defined as a nagging sense that something is missing, a lack of motivation, and a feeling of being "stuck" in a job or relationship.[4] When ignored, these conditions lead to insomnia, digestive problems, bad eating habits, addiction, depression, or emotional outbreaks. The results ring true. Recent statistics show that in the past two decades, there has been a 400 percent rise in the use of antidepressants for ages twelve and up.[5]

What causes this condition? Ellerby identified three factors, all of which are ways in which we lose touch with our inner spirit: the loss of time for artistic pursuits, a loss of community living, and a focus on the external versus the internal.

Have you experienced inspiration deficit? To reverse the symptoms of inspiration deficit disorder, invest in activities that allow self-expression and that free your spirit. Ask yourself which creative pursuits can feed your spirit. Instead of putting your spirit's desires on the bucket list, start to invest in things that make your heart sing. You have the courage to bravely jump into your spirit's calling.

Your Inner Muse-ic

Music has been a source of inspiration since ancient times. The word *music* comes from the Greek *mousike,* which means "relating to the muses."[6] According to Greek mythology, the nine Muses were daughters of the Earth mother, Gaia, and the god of the heavens, Uranus. You might say that creativity is the marriage of heaven and earth. Each of the nine muses inspired a branch of creativity and knowledge, from the arts to the sciences. Your muse-ic is the infinite creative potential, expressed in and through you as an awakened instrument.

Take a moment to remember your first joyous experience of music. It might be the first time that hearing a song touched your soul and made you want to sing along. It might be a moment with a parent's lullaby or with you banging on pots and pans on the floor of the kitchen. When did musical joy first awaken in you? Where were you when it happened? Doesn't it feel good to remember? This is the seed of your musical spirit.

The Art of Inner Music

Rich metaphors arise as we recognize that we are the music. We have a timbre, a unique sound quality reflected in the quality of our human experience. We have a vibration, a vibrancy felt when our inner music is playing in our hearts. We embody the inner music of each element in music's medicine and resonate through each principle.

Four Principles of Inner Music

1. *You Are Rhythm.* When you live in touch with your inner rhythm, every step is an embodied beat in the groove of life. We all have a biological beat, the heartbeat that is our inner drummer. At the close of my drum circles, I often ask people to put their hand over their hearts and repeat after me: "I am the drum of my heart."

George Leonard coined the term "silent pulse," referring to the invisible, artistic uniqueness in the rhythm of each person's unique spirit, expressed through music, writing, drama, dance, or visual arts. The pulse of creativity within may be "silent," but the arts give voice to our unique inner rhythm.

You embody the principle of rhythm—entrainment. Your spirit and your authentic groove affect those around you. You notice that people of similar rhythms are drawn to you, helping you express yourself more fully and effortlessly through a circle of support. Your individual rhythm allows others to embody their own authentic rhythms.

2. *Your Life Is Your Song.* We all compose unique melodies in our lives. Some of us explore a wide range of notes, venturing out into many new experiences, while others prefer to sing a repeated and simpler chant. Our individual melody is the contour, the themes and variations of the high and low notes, of our lives.

You embody the principle of melody; you possess a sonic alchemy. You become more sensitive to what you feed your ears. You choose songs that uplift, center, inspire, and free you. You recognize the effect of song on your heart and choose wisely what to sing and listen to. Your voice is resonant, your tone is clear, and you hold the capacity to "change your tune" when needed.

3. *You Are Harmony.* Your biology is filled with harmony: the balance of sleep and rest, the duet of body and spirit, and all the inner workings of health that are a concert of connections. Your soul is in harmony. Your relationships reverberate in harmony.

You embody the principle of harmony; you have a sympathetic vibration. Life begins to harmonize with you. Sometimes you are the dominant note, and sometimes you are the supporting note. Your inner harmony allows dissonance to seek resolution. Dissonant relationships gradually resolve or experience a *decrescendo,* softly fading away.

4. *You Rest in Silence.* Resting the mind, you allow more space for creative expression, free of mental fear, doubt, and worry. You consciously make space and hold space. You create space between the notes of your life, taking moments for contemplation and rest. Instead of a frenetic pace toward fast and furious cacophony, the music of your life breathes to honor the "peace-full-ness." Meaningful moments of shared silence occur between yourself and others. You become a master at using silence in speech and in musical expression. You enjoy the deep satisfaction of listening to musical silence.

You embody the principle of silence, of resting. The principle of resting allows you to balance and revive, to be recharged and available. You are present and peaceful, regularly clearing your mind and allowing spaciousness into your life.

The Creative Force of You

We develop musical skill by studying music written by a composer, but we develop our musical spirit through self-expression. You are the only one who can play the music that is uniquely your own. It is what makes Willie Nelson sound so different from Michael Jackson. The keys to creative expression lie in both composition and improvisation, and both have scientific evidence supporting their use in healing.

In his book *Inner Music*, Jamie Kassler said that the mind is the conductor, but the spirit is the composer.[7] When we compose music, we connect to the powerful spirit of creation. In the act of creating, we get to feel the essence of the Great Creator. Our motivation may vary from writing a song as a gift to honor a loved one to making up our own personal anthem. As we saw in Chapter 4, songwriting is an instinct; it is everyone's birthright. You are the composer of your own life's song.

Winging It

When we improvise—not only in music but also in any art form—we say we are "winging it." Improvisation happens freely, spontaneously, "on the fly." Like a bird spreading its wings, we ride the ever-changing wind currents of creativity. But improvisation can be scary; we must leave the nest of written notes on a page and soar with the voice from within our musical spirit.

When you improvise, you move from learning music written in the past to creating music in the now. It is unrehearsed, spontaneous, and driven by your musical spirit. It is a jam session, a tool of conversation between human instruments. As we'll see in the research, you cannot force this type of musical expressiveness. It is bred in the fertile ground of permission, not performance; and it comes from creativity, not complexity.

The Principle of Inner Music—Resonant Frequency

When something feels right with our inner spirit, we say it resonates or rings true. Resonance is the reverberation of truth. *Resonance* means "a rich sound; a lasting presence or effect."[8]

Resonance is the audible equivalent of radiance. We are familiar with radiance, a quality of a person whose spirit is bright and light. Resonance is the sonic essence expressed in a person's energy. Resonance is felt in presence.

In musical acoustics, the note that most reverberates is called *resonant frequency*. When you sing across a drum, you hear the tone that resonates the membrane. By playing around through scales of notes, you suddenly hear a resonance that amplifies and creates an echo, a reverberation. You've discovered the instrument's core pitch.

We also have a resonant pitch that rings from our inner spirit. Acoustic chambers create the space that brings out resonance; this is why we sound good when singing in the shower or why a choir singing in a spacious cathedral sounds so wonderful. There is also an inner chamber that supports the expression of our resonance, a spaciousness that allows a note to resonate. By holding space and being open, there is a greater resonance of our inner tonality.

The Science of Inner Music

A recent study compared improvisation with playing memorized music and found surprising results. Our brains show that improvisation is an expression of our deepest individual personality. Perhaps more importantly, the jazz of "winging it" disengages the self-monitoring that can bind our creativity. Again, it is a pattern of what music *undoes* that creates the healing space for the inner musical spirit.

Permission, Not Perfection

Charles Limb is a surgeon and jazz pianist who studies the way musical creativity works in the brain. He is on the faculty of both the Johns Hopkins School of Medicine and the Peabody Conservatory of Music. He developed his research at the National Institutes of Health.

In a study using functional magnetic resonance imagining (fMRI) to look at brain activity, Limb compared two music-making conditions with jazz musicians: playing a memorized composition versus improvising music, where the musicians made up their own solos. His research team used a small plastic piano with thirty-five keys, as opposed to a full eighty-eight-key piano—because it fit inside the fMRI machine.

The results showed that only when musicians improvised did a very specific, small area of the brain's frontal cortex—the medial prefrontal cortex—become activated. This same area functions in self-reflection, intro-spection, personal sharing, and self-expression; it is often thought to be the seat of consciousness. This part of the brain is activated when we talk about ourselves, telling our personal story. When they were improvising, the musicians were revealing their true identities, their musical spirits. No two improvised jazz pieces were the same.

Simultaneously, a deactivation occurred during improvisation. Two larger areas of the frontal cortex—the lateral prefrontal cortex and the dorsolateral prefrontal cortex—were deactivated. These areas deal with self-monitoring, judgment, and self-criticism. The brain turns off the self-monitoring and inhibitory judgment in order to access the uniqueness of our individual cre-ativity. With a willingness to make mistakes, the mind removes self-judgment in order to free up more expression of the true authentic spirit of each player. The jazz brain is a palette of permission, not perfection.[9]

No wonder courageous self-expression in the arts is a battle. The larger parts of the brain inhibit our self-expression, while the smaller part reveals the greater self.

Creativity, Not Complexity

In a second phase of the study, Limb removed the element of musician-ship in order to test the pure spirit of creativity without complexity. He restricted the playing of the jazz pianists by only allowing them to improvise from an eight-note scale and to only play on the downbeats. He compared this type of limited improvisation to a fuller expression of twelve-bar blues, in which the musicians once again improvised freely. Amazingly, the brain imaging showed that whether playing complex rhythms or fancy notes, the same results occurred—the same areas were activated and deactivated. It's the creativity, not the complexity, that puts us in the jazz state of mind.

Whether you are a trained pianist or someone who has never played an instrument before, there is a path to improvisation, a way of expressing music, that is completely and uniquely your own—a sonic fingerprint. I have always felt that improvisation should be the way we begin music education. Why wait to read notes when the notes are already written in our musical spirit?

Creative Music Therapy

The Nordoff-Robbins Center for Music Therapy in New York has been demonstrating that even those children with great emotional or physical challenges and disabilities have a song to play. Founded in 1961 through a partnership between composer Paul Nordoff and special education teacher Clive Robbins, the center currently treats children with cerebral palsy, autism, Asperger's disease, and others with developmental delays. The center's approach to healing is entirely based on a belief in the musical spirit within every child. Robbins said, "Our mission is to transform lives through music; to reach each child's developmental potential."

Music therapist Kenneth Aigen described the Nordoff-Robbins improvisational technique and how it supports each client's inner musical expression. First, the music therapist matches the sound environment to the client's inner self, noticing which sounds resonate and attract the child. Second, the therapist creates a musical environment in which the client can naturally express him- or herself. The music experiences and the joy of self-expression translate into real-life skills: more self-expression, improved mood, and increased social interactions. According to Aigen, "There are intrinsic psychological and spiritual benefits within the creation of music."[10]

A study from the Institute of Neuropalliative Rehabilitation in London showed the importance of creative music therapy based on improvisation in adults with chronic mental illnesses. Music therapy researchers found that improvisation provides a positive sense of identity, which enables a dramatic shift from disempowerment to empowerment. Improvisation also allows active participation and a sense of control, skill, and success. These are strong healing attributes that are much needed when facing chronic illnesses such as depression and bipolar disorder.[11]

Composing Is Healing

Why have we come to assume that only a select few can write songs? In music therapy, songwriting is a proven tool for personal transformation and healing.

No prior musical training is required. When we write a song or create an improvisation, we realize that the medicine of our healing is within us.

In a large survey of almost five hundred music therapists from twenty-nine countries, researchers found common themes of the benefits of songwriting as a tool of healing. Clients showed measured improvement in self-confidence, a sense of mastery, an improved sense of self, the ability to express their story, and a demonstration of insights into thoughts and feelings.[12]

In summary, improvisation and composition are tributaries of the out-pouring flow of musical spirit within us, an expression of our unique musical spirit and our authentic personality. The conditions of permission not performance, creativity not complexity, and improvisation not memorization are all part of the formula of the science of inner music.

The Spirit of Inner Music

Sound is a portal into the inner temple. Gurus, Sufis, yogis, and mystics have long described the spiritual path of awakening in terms of sound. Chanting, toning, and sounding the names of the Divine are ways to create communion and union with the divine vibration. Invisible, yet audible, this vibration is believed to be a pathway into the interior realms where spirit resides singing.

In the Hindu writings of the Upanishads, *ohm* is the sound of the birthing of the universe. The three sounds of "a-u-m" combined represent the union of the three Gods—Vishnu, Shiva, and Brahma—a trinity in sound. Lorin Roche, PhD, shares a simple translation, distilling the rich complexity in Sanskrit. According to Roche, *ohm* means "yes"—also thought of as "the roar of joy."[13] Imagine that roar of joy humming within you. Yum.

In Sant Mat, the ancient path of saints from India introduced to me by Connor Sauer, the term *shabd* refers to the eternal sound current, the "audible life stream."[14] In deep inner listening, devotees report specific sounds in the inner realms: wind blowing, thunder, waves of the ocean, bells, drums, celestial harmonies, and silence. *The Radiance Sutras* describe similar sounds of hand bells, flutes, strings, and the buzzing of bees.[15] To awaken to these inner sounds, devotees chant mantras, and sing melodies of kirtan or bhajan style; but they also tune out the external world to tune into the inner realms.

In the Christian tradition, the invisible vibratory presence is referred to as the Holy Ghost, or the fire that anointed the speaking of tongues on the day of Pentecost. In my time playing piano at the Soul Saving Station for Every Nation in New York, I experienced this ritual of Holy Spirit anointing and witnessed many church members going into a free expression of sounding, dancing, weeping, and healing through speaking in tongues.

Working in the Middle East, I experienced *tarab,* a state of spiritual ecstasy through music that is felt when the presence of Spirit takes over the performance, igniting everyone in attendance—musicians and audience alike. As a young Arab woman explained to me, "The musicians are talking to Allah." It seems there is a universal spiritual understanding of a sound current of the Divine that is accessed through music and tapped from within.

Tuning In

How do we tune into the sound current that is within? We turn our attention away from the outer realms and into the sound of our inner spirit. It may take closing our eyes, plugging our ears, closing off the external to hear the inner sound. Sutra 91 of *The Radiance Sutras* (translated by Lorin Roche) offers a poetic path into the inner music:

> Close the ears that track the outer world
> Open the ears of the soul
> The song of creation, the unstruck chord,
> Is playing in your heart . . .
> Listen in.
> Meditating on the sound of your own life currents,
> Enter the shimmering palace of the Creator.[16]

Be Your Note

You have a pitch, a note, a fundamental vibration of your inner spirit that is uniquely your own. Just as musicians with a good ear have perfect pitch, I call the inner pitch your *personal pitch*. It is the note of you.

You may notice that when you are around a resonant person, his or her vibration is different from that of someone who is upset and angry. You may notice that the pitch of an upbeat person is filled with joy and celebration; this is different from the note of someone who is feeling depressed and self-criticizing. Rumi captured this essence in poetry, as translated by Coleman Barks:

God picks up the reed-flute world and blows.
Each note is a need coming through one of us,
a passion, a longing-pain . . .
Sing loud.[17]

Attunement

Although you may be familiar with the tantric tradition, you may not know what
a music metaphor this term really is. The Sanskrit term *tantra* comes from *tantri*,
meaning "to tune."[18] Inner tuning involves the strings of the heart, the chords of
the soul, and the rhythm of the body in creating harmony; it means attunement.
When we are out of tune, like a musical instrument, our note falls flat; its sound
is deadened. Resonance is lost. Tuning is the process; resonance is the result.

Be in Tune

Before entering the symphony of life, we must first tune ourselves. Musicians
call this intonation, or intoning the most resonant sound. For some people,
tuning occurs through meditation every morning. For others, it is a morning ritual. My grandfather used to read the spiritual guide "The Daily
Bread" every morning before breakfast. It was his tuning process, the way
he attuned himself spiritually and tuned himself mentally. I've included a
simple morning attunement exercise in the guided practices (page 150) to
support your daily tune-up.

Being in tune is an ongoing process. During the course of a concert,
as the temperature rises from the bright lights, you see performers retun-
ing their instruments to adjust to this change. The outer environment can
throw off our tuning throughout the day. Frequent check-ins and adjust-
ments, inner listening, and recalibration of ourselves help keep us in tune.
This tune-up can be done in sacred moments alone, through deep breathing,
or even by sitting in silence. It may be done as a toning practice, like the
exercise included in the guided practices.

You can't tune someone else's instrument. Even though you can hear
when others are out of tune, they are the only ones who can correct their
intonation. It is each person's responsibility to maintain the tuning of his or
her own instrument.

What are the signs that you are out of tune? How do you recalibrate
your inner song? In life, we may be pulled off pitch, causing us to become

sharp or flat by circumstances that may tighten or loosen our inner note and change our resonance. However, like the purity of the sound of a tuning fork, you can feel when you are back in tune with your inner pitch. Think about what retunes you and how you can maintain your perfect pitch.

The Medicine of Inner Music—Resonance

There is healing in discovering the medicine of the inner music. So often, in the face of illness or tragedy, we dig deeper to discover its song.

I was working with a young woman who was a survivor of early childhood abuse. Therapists viewed her as resistant because she wouldn't talk, so she was referred to music therapy. When she first arrived, she immediately went to the drum set. It seemed to resonate with her spirit. As she grew more comfortable with me and with the drums, she became gradually more expressive of her emotions through creative improvisation. When she was ready, I guided her in a music experience of telling her story of abuse through the drum set, improvising and composing her own music.

For twenty minutes, she became lost in the playing while I recorded her music. When we listened to the playback, she smiled, hearing her strength pounding on the drums and her creative rhythms. She felt proud and empowered and successful in her own self-expression. She had moved from resistance to resonance.

Recognizing that we are instruments for expressing the music within us can have effects beyond our own healing to create change in the world. This was the case for Rick Allen, the drummer for Def Leppard. I interviewed Rick in 2002 for an article on rhythms of renewal for a drum magazine.

In 1984, at the age of nineteen, Rick was at the height of his rock-and-roll drum career when he lost his left arm in a car accident. Waking up in the hospital bed, he was told he would never drum again. Rick gave up hope until one day something magical happened.

Rick told me, "In my first week in the hospital, I started hearing music that just seemed to be playing. I thought it was coming out of the air vents. But it was coming from me, from a place within me. I told my brother to go home and get the stereo system and my music collection. I started listening to my favorite music: Led Zeppelin, Free, Bad Company, T-Rex, David Bowie."

Just listening helped his mood tremendously. His brother also brought drumsticks and a practice pad, which sat untouched in the corner of the room. Then one day, while listening to the music, Rick noticed that his feet were unconsciously tapping to the beat. "I suddenly realized that the music was not in my arms; it was in *me*. I just had to figure out a new way to get it out."

The rest of the story is well known in rock-music circles. Rick began the hard work of reassigning drumbeats he'd always played with his left arm to his right arm and both legs. He designed a custom drum set with electronic foot pedals. Within a few months, he was onstage, performing in front of fifty-five thousand screaming fans, reunited with his musical spirit and the band.

But the story didn't end there. Not only did Rick reclaim his music, he also became an instrument of healing veterans through drum circles, launching his organization Raven Drum Foundation with partner Lauren Monroe. In 2002, Rick was honored with a Humanitarian Award in California. Through his organization, Rick now revives the rhythms in wounded warriors through resiliency programs.[19] Find out more at ravendrumfoundation.com. For the full article on Rick, see ubdrumcircles.com/article_rhythm.html.

Final Chorus

We are all instruments, incubated in rhythm, born in melody, matured through harmony, and resting in silence. We are *musica humana*—musical spirits. Yet, as in music, it is not the instrument that makes sound. Even the most beautifully tuned instrument is silent until played. It is the unique voice of our spirit, brought forth in the tributaries of self-expression, improvisation, composition, and the creative sounding of our spirit, that makes music.

There is a reason we say we "play" music. Notes want to be played, rhythms want to be danced, harmonies want to resonate, and silence wants room to breathe. Embody this inner musical spirit and be strong in your note, resonant in your vibration, and present in your pitch.

As in life, inner discovery is a journey filled with challenges that can pull us away from the inner self. We become inspiration-deprived and out of breath in the attempt to keep up with life's outer demands. Yet here in the center of our spirit is a song, a rhythm, harmony, and silence awaiting discovery and expression.

GUIDED PRACTICES FOR THE
MEDICINE OF INNER MUSIC

These practices are designed to tune and attune your human instrument and empower the inner music that is the resonance of your spirit. Where do you need more spirit, a sense of inspiration, or greater self-expression in your life? Has a part of you been reborn in the process of reading this book? Is there a new awareness of the four healing elements of music medicine that are within you?

These conscious listening and expressing practices are designed to awaken your musical spirit. The playlist features voice and drums, two innate sounds in the human instrument, like our heartbeat and vocal strings. It is filled with opportunities for you to sound your spirit; to sing and drum; and to create, improvise, and compose. Follow what resonates with you as you dive into the inner realms of your own creative spirit.

Guided Practices for Conscious Listening

Listening to Your Inner Music

As a human instrument, you are the first track on the inner-music playlist. Consider this a meditation on the four elements of music reverberating within you. Take a few deep breaths. Clear your mind. With awakened ears and a resonant heart, enter this journey into musical awakening.

Listen to the rhythm in your body. It is the forward motion of life's pulsing heartbeat. This is the medicine for your body. Place your fingers on your pulse and feel your inner rhythm. Hear your breath combine with the rhythm of your heart in a polyrhythm of aliveness. Feel that you are the walking, talking, tick-tocking rhythm of life. Sense the rhythm of your own body expressing its beat. Celebrate your unique dance of rhythmical freedom.

Listen to the melody in your heart. Every day offers an opportunity to sing a new song. Your heart resonates with all your favorite songs and strongest power songs. Feel your heartstrings vibrating. Listen to the melody within you, the vibration and tone that are you.

Listen to the harmony of your soul. Sense how life wants to harmonize. Feel the ensemble of your body and mind singing, drumming, and being fully present and alive. Harmonize with all of life, knowing that you belong here now. Feel at ease with nature's beauty; be compassionate and connected. Sense the music bridge between yourself and all others. You are in a constant duet with the planet, nature, animals, and humanity. Harmonize your inner music with the ensemble of life.

Listen to the silence of your mind. Imagine the silence that makes space between the notes of your life and that opens sonic doorways to inner peace. Feel the silence deep within your own being, a sense of peaceful, calm resting; enjoy a moment of pause and contemplation. Hear all sounds around you, while also listening intently to the silence between them. Allow the inner silence to be the empty place of ethereal contact. Breathe deeply and rest in the stillness. Enter the music of silence.

Turn within, to the Center, where the inner music of your spirit is playing. Hear all the elements of rhythm, melody, harmony, and silence singing through you and as you—singing in the rhythm of your body, the song of your heart, the harmony between your body and soul, and the peace of inner silence. Become more and more of your authentic sound, note by note and beat by beat. Become a human instrument; feel the creativity of your inner music that only you can play.

Ear Training

As you develop your spirit ears, notice what you listen to in life. What resonates with you? What sound grabs your attention? Do you listen more to criticism or encouragement? Do you tune into fear or freedom, worry or wonder, dissonance or resonance? When you need inspiration, activate your spirit ears and listen for the good. It's what musicians call "ear training." Instead of the cacophony of life, hear the music. It might be a positive comment from a friend or workmate or the sound of wind blowing in a forest through the trees. Develop a practice of hearing the beauty, and notice how your musical spirit dances in the positive vibration it loves to hear.

With your spirit ears, listen to music you love, or start with the inner-music playlist. Let the music reach into your inner spirit. Be open. Music travels into the places of our open spirit, like water flows into open ponds.

Make Me an Instrument

(Tracks 2, 4, 5, and 9 from the online inner-music playlist)
Listen deeply to the resonant voices of Laurel Massé of Manhattan Transfer

(track 4) and Silvia Nakkach (track 5). Hear the quality of tone and voice that is pure, centered, and reverberant. There is no language in the spirit voice, only sound, syllable, and pure expression.

Track 2 reminds you that you are rhythm; the soft heartbeat that plays throughout the drum improvisation is like your body's beat. Listen to and feel your inner rhythmical spirit awakening. Track 9 is composed purely of rhythm and voice. Master drummer Glen Velez uses rhythmic vocalization in the Indian tradition—"Ta–Ka–Di–Mi" and "Dum–Pa–Za." As you listen, feel an activation of your own rhythm and voice.

Invoking Your Muse

(Track 4)

Awakening the inner musical spirit just takes an invitation. We don't have to beg for creativity to appear in our lives; we just call to our muse or chant it alive in our lives. Awakening the inner musical spirit is how we invoke the muse that creates the inspiration to evoke our musical expression. This recording is an ancient Greek chant to the muse of the beautiful voice. Imagine your inner muse receiving the call.

Guided Practices for Expressing

Ohm

(Track 1)

I can think of no better way to begin than by toning *ohm*—the Sanskrit "yes"—and activating the "roar of joy" within you. Listen to or join Chloë Goodchild, founder of The Naked Voice, using the three distinct syllables: "ah," "ooo," and "mmm" that create *ohm*.

Begin by listening to the music—take a few deep, slow breaths and receive the sound in your inner spirit. As you breathe, become present to this moment. When you are ready, take a deep, belly breath to support your sound and then join the toning practice. Sustain your tone as long as you can; breathe when needed. Take time in between each note for silence. Let your spirit breathe. If an area of your body, mind, spirit, heart, or soul needs resonance, send the sound there. Surrender yourself into the sea of sound and float in the buoyancy of the universal hum.

Morning Attunement

(Track 5)

Each day is a new opportunity to be part of the music of life. When you start the day with music, you awaken more than your body; your spirit becomes alive in sound. Sounding your spirit, you unify with the vibration of creativity.

If you've read *The Artist's Way* by Julia Cameron, you've experienced the power of her morning-pages practice. Similarly, you can start the day with a morning music practice of your own creative design, which may change or unfold like a musical improvisation. Begin with intention. I like to face east to connect with the direction of the new day, new rhythm, and new song. You may want to hum, sing, chant, or drum. You may have a mantra or affirmation that expresses your feeling of connection with the Divine.

If you like to drum, start the day with an improvised drumbeat, an expression of your rhythmical spirit. No words are needed but if you prefer to use language in sound, consider an affirmation that can be slowly chanted and repeated. It may also be words that describe your inner spirit. Be like the birds that herald a new day by singing in the forest. Awaken the sense that you are the music and that life today will be the next movement in your life's symphony of love, joy, and creativity.

Toning Your Note

As you go through the day, there will be moments that knock you out of tune; dissonance will arise, and inner strings can tighten and sometimes even break. Any time you need to retune yourself throughout the day, use this simple practice of toning your note. Toning comes from "tone," just the single note that is an inner sounding.

Just as a note sounds more resonant in an open space, take a moment and imagine the spaciousness around your inner spirit. Envision that your spirit lives in a circular chamber or an open cathedral. Give yourself permission to sing your note, whatever it may be, and let it resonate your whole being.

This practice is surprisingly natural—I've done this for years with hundreds of people. Trust yourself. Be your note. Sing loud.

When you complete the toning of your note, allow time to sit with the vibration. Allow the note to settle you. Receive what a beautiful spirit you are, what a clear, resonant essence you have.

Toning Your Energy Centers

(Track 6)

Traditional Chinese medicine states that each organ has a pitch, a note. Imagine that your whole inner body is a network of notes in harmony. To activate the physical body song, hum or tone a note and notice where you feel it in your body. Try a lower or higher note and see how it changes. Can you sing into your belly? Your heart? Your throat? Your mind? Notice the places where you are too tight and see if you can resonate your body with sound.

Toning can also be used to harmonize and tune energy centers that are beyond the physical. These chakra points have sounds that vary according to different world traditions. In the tradition of Vedic chakras, the sounds are *lang, vang, rang, yang, hang,* and *ohm*. The recording "Elements into Light" (track 6) introduces you to a toning practice, in the key of B, that uses these syllables and that is a good overall tuning.

Expressing Your Musical Spirit

(Tracks 7 and 8)

You have a unique creative spirit—a song and rhythm that only you can play. Improvisation is a great tool of personal growth and healing that can also free your spirit to be more fully alive. Using a drum or voice or any instrument you choose, get ready to improvise and make up your own music to these backing tracks.

As you start to listen to the music, begin by anchoring yourself in your first memory of musical joy. Remember a time when you were touched by sound, a joyful moment of musical connection. Bring that energy into this practice now. Remember that the key to improvisation is creativity not complexity, permission not perfection. In creative improvisation, there are no wrong notes.

When you play along with a backing track, it can be helpful to use headphones. To balance hearing yourself and the track, you can try moving one side of the headphones off your ear slightly. Always give yourself at least four minutes to fall into the music and begin to open up to your own creativity. Both tracks are long enough to allow you to take your time.

Track 7 is an instrumental groove in the key of E for your rhythm spirit, expressed on a drum or with body percussion. You may want to begin by joining the pulse of the music and then gradually develop your own magic.

Track 8 is a spacious palette for your vocal improvisation, also in the key of E. Use a vowel sound like "ah" or a scatting syllable like "hey ya," and let yourself jam along with the music. When you finish, receive the inner applause clapping for your creative freedom.

ANNOTATED PLAYLIST
FOR INNER MUSIC
••••••••••••••••••

To stream this music, visit SoundsTrue.com/MusicMedicine.

1. "Aum," Chloë Goodchild, *Your Naked Voice*
Ah-ooo-mmm is clearly annunciated in the three syllables to the
note A, a common pitch of tuning. For more on Chloë Goodchild, visit
thenakedvoice.com or consider delving into The Naked Voice audio course.

2. "Return Journey," Randy Crafton, *Inner Rhythms*
Master drummer Randy Crafton jams to the primal heartbeat that is softly
playing in the background. Rhythm is what we are made of, and this recording takes us into the inner realms of our entire being in perfect timing—the
polyrhythm of heart beating, lungs breathing, and cells vibrating.

3. "Kerala Dream," Shaman's Dream, *Kerala Dream*
It is often said that we are dreaming ourselves awake. What is real, and what is
the dream? Fall into the reality of the inner music in this watery composition
filled with the call of the flute, an expression of improvised musical spirit.

4. "Hymn to the Muse," Layne Redmond and Laurel Massé,
Invoking the Muse
This ancient chant, written on Crete around 120 BCE, calls to the golden
Greek muse of beautiful voice: "O muse, precious one, sing to me, Thy
inspiration a prelude for my own song. Inspire my heart and mind." Sung by
Laurel Massé, of Manhattan Transfer fame, with Layne Redmond on drums.

5. "Morning Melody," Silvia Nakkach, *Medicine Melodies*
Greet the day with the voice that rises like the sunlight from deep within our
spirit. Sense your own musical spirit rising over David Darling's beautiful cello.
Free Your Voice, a great new book by Silvia Nakkach, can help you liberate your
musical spirit.

6. "Elements into Light," Layne Redmond, *Chanting the Chakras: Roots of Awakening*
This piece focuses on chanting the six chakra seed syllables around the tonal pitch of B:
Lang: root from feet to knees
Vang: base of spine
Rang: heart
Yang: center of head
Hang: crown
Aum: to the highest point of Divine light

7. "Breath of the Chakras: Instrumental Version," Layne Redmond, *Chakra Breathing Meditations*
Featuring frame drums, Tibetan singing bowls, bells, chimes, and tamboura, this track carries a rhythm journey for play-along in the key of E or for chanting your own spirit voice. A very gradual tempo that increases throughout the piece brings an invitation for greater creative freedom. This track is long enough for you to really get into it and let your own rhythm and voice be expressed. Let go and join the sound.

8. "Shamanic Journey Berimbau Rhythm," Hank Wesselman and Jill Kuykendall, *Sound Journeys: Compiled by Sandra Ingerman*
Sound is the carrier wave into the shamanic portal of the inner self. The pulse of a *clave*—or two wooden sticks tapped together—accompanies the rattle and *berimbau,* a Brazilian single-stringed, bowlike instrument with a gourd to resonate the sound. Listen to the harmonic overtones of the string. This track is long, designed for you to join in and discover your musical spirit, chant your own spirit song, or add your own drum or percussion.

9. "Farewell Wave," Glen Velez, *Breathing Rhythms*
This track is a great demonstration of the human instrument—voice and percussion. Master drummer Glen Velez combines voicing rhythmic syllables "Ta–Ka–Di–Mi" and "Dum–Pa–Za" to the beat played on a *riq,* low- and high-pitched cardboard boxes, a *bodhrán* frame drum from Ireland, a *pandeiro,* a cello, and a pan flute.

8

Orchestrating Change: Medicine for the World

From a distance we are instruments
Marching in a common bond.
Playing songs of hope, playing songs of peace.
They're the songs of every man.

—JULIE GOLD, "FROM A DISTANCE"

I n Iraq, with no translators in sight, we sometimes had to resort to musical communication. Someone would approach us during a break, and unable to find a translator, he or she would just break into clapping rhythms to talk to us. We'd all laugh and join in the language of rhythm until a translator could be found. This type of thing began to happen over and over—at lunch with tableware and in the hotel lobby, where someone would start singing and we'd tap along using body percussion. No translator needed.

When the program ended, I wondered how the joy-filled, peaceful energy would extend into their lives and mine. About a month after I returned home, an instant message popped up on my computer screen. It looked like someone had closed their eyes and typed random keys on the computer; it was completely illegible. I wrote back a question mark. The response was, "No English." And then, "Jihad."

Jihad was a talented violinist from Halabja, Iraq, the place of the worst chemical-warfare genocide in history, where Saddam Hussein's Anvil Regime killed more than five thousand Kurds in one day. Jihad was one of our best drum-circle leaders, who played his violin to add melody to the peace-building drum circles.

There was no sense in writing back in English, so I typed back using the language of the drum: "doum doum tak-a-tak." "Doum" (usually written "dum") and "tak" (pronounced "taak") are, respectively, the main onomato-poeic tones of the low and high sounds on the Middle Eastern drum. Jihad knew what I meant. He replied, "Doum doum tak-a tak tak."

I typed back "doum doum," like the lub–dub of a heartbeat, and hit send. I waited, giving pause between the beats, and then wrote again, "doum doum." He understood my heartbeat and echoed back, "doum doum." We were doing call-and-response, sharing heartfelt communication that was beyond words in the sonic lexicon we both spoke fluently.

Jihad's next message was an attachment of a sound file of him playing violin. We had moved into melody. As I listened to the short music clip, I felt like I was right there next to him, instead of thousands of miles away and oceans apart. I wondered if this could be the future of digital dialogue in the universal language of music. What followed was "*zor supas*," which is Kurdish for "thank you." Then the connection was lost—or was it?

The following year, I returned to Iraq. The danger was beginning to lessen, and our sponsors invited us to travel to Halabja, where, in a town filled with mass graves, Jihad was leading drum circles in schools and youth centers. He was playing his violin to the traumatized hearts of his beloved community; his musical service was working. While I was there, in a drum circle that he led with a large group of young people, everyone started chanting, "Halabja is alive! Halabja is alive!"

After the program, I sat outside with Jihad, waiting for the others so we could all walk together to a lunch café. As if we never missed a beat, we began talking in "doum-tak-tak-doum doum" back and forth. After a few minutes of dialogue, Jihad smiled and ended our musical conversation with "doum-doum," tapping his hand over his heart to the beat.

The Global Language

I believe that music is a key tool for transformation on the planet, ushering in a time of harmony in our new co-created world. We are witnessing more and more musicians becoming activists—or as some say, "artivists"—performers who are becoming reformers.

It's ironic that language, which developed for communication, can be a barrier to global connection. At the edge of words, we find there is so much more to say to one another, so much more to express of our souls than just our thoughts. In today's world of increasing connectivity and an ever-more expansive global perspective, we need a universal language to create the dialogues of the future; we need a language of the soul. The music bridge of harmony applies to global peace building. We are living in the stage of harmony on the planet, birthing a world that works for all of us.

Real change cannot come by words alone—or by music alone, for that matter. I'm not a believer in the "Kumbaya" approach to global conflict. It's the combination of both music and words that builds relationships and allows honest dialogue to flow—an extension of the soul-to-soul connection between people who make music together.

Music gives us creative citizenship in the world we all belong to. That world is changing and finding more and more ways to harmonize. In a global perspective, harmony is the stage of music's medicine happening in the world today. We have seen lots of drumming and singing around the world, but it's the harmony of collaboration and relationships that is being birthed today. Even in our relationship with nature, we have the opportunity to live in greater harmony through music's medicine. Together, we can share in the elevation and evolution of the planetary song.

The Art of Orchestrating Change

In the movie *Ten Questions for the Dalai Lama,* His Holiness is asked what we can do to create peace. With a huge smile on his face, the Dalai Lama says: "More music festivals."[1]

There is a rise in the number of world music concerts and festivals of cultural sharing. It's rare to find a peace conference that doesn't include some musical component. The feeling tone of a performer playing for peace reaches our hearts, even when we don't understand the words.

Have you ever heard live music in another language and felt a connection to the sound, even without understanding the meaning? If so, you have experienced the universal feeling tone that underlies the music.

Performers Becoming Reformers

A sign that we are orchestrating change is the growing ensembles of performers using music to awaken hearts, unify audiences, communicate a message of hope, and empower survivors of violence. Together, they create inspiration, hope, and transformation. Singing and performing in places of great conflict and despair, these reformers are laying down the tracks of the new song lines into the grid of transformation.

Many immediately think of Bono, from the rock group U2, and for good reason. He was awarded the distinction "Man of Peace" by the Nobel Laureates in 2008, he was nominated for a Nobel Peace Prize, and he has worked to raise awareness of global poverty for more than two decades. In a historic partnership with YouTube, the U2 concert at the Pasadena Rose Bowl was broadcast live, allowing more than ten million viewers worldwide to sing together simultaneously. It became the largest streaming event on YouTube, but it was much more than that: I would say it was the largest musical peace rally to date.

In Bono's homeland of Dublin, Northern Ireland, with its long history of religious conflict, vocalist Chloë Goodchild of The Naked Voice (thenakedvoice.com) joined the Dalai Lama in singing and chanting for peace, the same place where the sounds of American folk singer Joan Baez still linger since she marched and sang there in 1978.

Michael Franti, founder of reggae group Spearhead, armed with a guitar and a compassionate heart, traveled to Iraq, Israel, and Palestine in 2004. His journey inspired the creation of the DVD *I Know I'm Not Alone* (iknowimnotalone.com). In his concerts, he tells stories of his experiences, bringing to American audiences a profound sense of a deeper purpose of music.

In an act of musical bravery, Kristina Sophia and Cameron Powers, from Musical Missions of Peace (musicalmissionsofpeace.org), sang Iraqi love songs on the streets of Baghdad at the start of the American occupation in 2003, as highlighted in their DVD *Singing in Baghdad*. True bridge builders, they traveled to the Middle East to learn love songs and carried the songs back to their performances in America. They have given hundreds of concerts across the United States and have performed in front of thousands in Egypt. One of their most amazing experiences was literally singing their way across the Iraqi border, where guards were so moved by their renditions of Arabic music that they allowed them to enter the country without visas. Talk about the global passport of music.

Afghani singer and songwriter Farhad Darya, a goodwill ambassador to the United Nations, has been uniting audiences, raising money for orphans, creating education for street children, and singing in places of suffering. In 2010, he created a concert for fifteen thousand Afghani women and girls. He performed the concert at a former Taliban headquarters, where many people, especially women, had been executed. If you Google him, you'll be inspired by his music videos (which have English subtitles), like "Brother," where he invites us to "sing along with me; without formality of languages, just like the bird canary." To learn more, visit daryasworld.com. At the edge of words, music is the transcendent language of the soul.

The transformation from performer to reformer involves four key paradigm shifts.

1. A performer plays an instrument; *a reformer becomes an instrument.*

2. A performer gets applause; *a reformer gives applause.*

3. A performer uses talent to be a success; *a reformer uses talent to make a difference.*

4. A performer entertains an audience; *a reformer transforms a community and even the world.*

Personally, I have been deeply transformed in the process of working in other countries and with other cultures. For years, I was a *go-getter,* full of ambition, aspiration, drive, and ego. By giving my musical gifts, I became a *go-giver,* touched at the core of my being by the powerful connections created through music medicine. Singing out for truth or traveling to places of conflict does not come without risk, but the rewards far outweigh any possibility of danger. Whenever we give, we receive so much more.

The Shadow Side of Orchestrating Change

Musical peacemaking efforts come with great risk. Artists are exiled, silenced, or, in the case of John Lennon, tragically killed for the beliefs they uphold in their music. Yet, despite the risk, the music does not die. The great Russian cellist Mstislav Rostropovich was exiled from his country for more than twenty years for speaking out against the Soviet Union's restriction of cultural freedom. He found refuge in the United States, joined the U.S. National Symphony Orchestra, and eventually gave a historic impromptu concert during the fall of the Berlin Wall.

The Science of Orchestrating Change

What is the effect of these inspiring stories of musical transformation? How do you measure success or evaluate changes in the hearts and souls of people experiencing music together?

Drum Dialogue

In the Ashti Drum project in Iraq in 2007—even though the forty-person training group represented different tribal, ethnic, and religious groups, making verbal communication impossible—we believed the musical communication would be healing on a personal level and transformative on a group level, with real, measurable benefits.

For this pilot project, I used subjective surveys, translated into both Kurdish and Arabic, before and after the five-day training program. We tested two measures: level of satisfaction with the drum-circle training and level of connection to one another. The group gave the training program a 92 percent satisfaction rating, a remarkably high score compared with other types of peacemaking efforts involving such divergent groups. I was also curious whether a real sense of community could occur within the group, despite their differences. Surprisingly, at the conclusion of the training, the group rated themselves at a level of 80 percent connected to their fellow trainees. The barriers of language, history, and war could be overcome through music.[2]

In addition to quantitative measures, I wanted to track some qualitative responses. On the final day of the training, I sat with two translators and conducted interviews with a randomly selected portion of the group. Holding back tears while operating a tape recorder and microphone, I listened to their statements:

"I was amazed to see people of different cultures making music together," said a chief from Mosul. "Drumming helps you find your hope," said a young Assyrian Christian woman. "The drum circle was the first time I could let go of my grief," said a Kurdish man whose mother was killed by Hussein's regime. "I never realized the power of people making music together. This program has been the best five days of my life," said an Arabic university student.

In the words of a director of Kurdistan Save the Children (KSC), "The drums create a new way of talking to each other. Through drum circles, we will bring more people together."[3] For more information on the Ashti Drum project, visit ashtidrum.com. For the full article on the project, visit ubdrumcircles.com/article_iraqi.html.

Real-World Results

Extending the drum-circle training into each facilitator's community was the ultimate evaluation of the program. Unfortunately, drum circles in the southern Arab part of Iraq were riskier and faced greater challenges and restrictions. However, in northern Iraq, with our partner KSC, drum circles started at four youth activity centers. They also started in a children's rehabilitation center and at a women's shelter, and they were woven into performances by a Kurdish drum ensemble playing the traditional *daf,* the drum of northern Iraq. In the town of Halabja, one of the worst places of genocide, the drum circles have been extended into schools to reach more children.

In the ancient land known as the birthplace of civilization, these facilitators are transforming drums of war into drums of peace. Their rhythms are being woven into the hearts of the next generation of youth, who are bringing hope, creativity, and collaboration to the healing of their culture and to the land that has suffered great tragedy and destruction. Healing is the much-needed outcome.

Song Lines

The Aboriginal people of Australia hold a belief that all land is sacred, and they must continually sing to it. Their culture believes in song lines that were woven into the land and sky by creator beings, such as Snake and Bird, who sang the name of every creature they encountered as they walked or flew. The creator beings sang the world alive while leaving footsteps and markers of their pathways. Songs are navigational tools across the bush and the interior desert lands; they are maps of the walkabout. A single song line may travel great distances through different tribal cultures, so the songs are sung in different languages along the walkabout journey. Yet somehow the melody shows the contour of the land, and the rhythm marks the footsteps. The songs guide the way.

I find this ancient tradition to be a useful metaphor for creating our new world in song. To me, song lines are being implanted today with each act of musical service, each opportunity to carry a message or musical tradition to another land.

The art of exchange is the music of the future. The concerts that are given and the performers who are traveling to inspire and unify us are the new song lines being woven around the world, even in the digital landscape of the virtual cosmos. Music creates a sonic matrix of peace.

Imagine the song lines of your life's journey as a human instrument, both as a metaphor and as an actual vibratory path.

What is the resonance of the music of your life? What kind of paths do you weave? If each step were a rhythm and each word were a melody, what is the kind of music in the song lines you are weaving?

The Medicine of Orchestrating Change

In the aftermath of tragedies, governments fund the costly process of reconstructing and rebuilding of infrastructures. Yet, how do we tend to the task of rebuilding the "inner structures" of the souls of people who are wounded by war or natural disasters? What tools reach the inner realms to help rebuild the soul?

In Japan, after World War II, music helped restore the spirit and cultural pride of Japanese people through government-supported Suzuki violin lessons. In Estonia, music brought tens of thousands of people together in football stadiums in what is considered "the singing revolution," which led to liberation from Soviet rule in 1991. In Brazil, in the *favelas* (slums), drug-trafficker-turned-revolutionary Anderson Sa inspired young people to resist through the lyrics of Afro-reggae music, inspiring the film *Favela Rising*. And in Uganda, music gave refugee children living in a war camp, who were more used to holding rifles than percussion mallets, a sense of family, beauty, and purpose. It became the first refugee camp to win a place in the Uganda National Music Competition, a story told in the documentary *War Dance*.

Transforming Poverty

One program that shows the power of music's medicine for cultural healing has to do with the fight against poverty in Latin America. Since 1975, the organization El Sistema has provided more than two million Venezuelan children with free music instruction. The program, created by musician and economist José Antonio Abreu, is aimed at reaching impoverished neighborhoods. It started with only twelve children and grew into the highly acclaimed Venezuelan Youth Orchestra.

Through free music education, the children become excellent musicians and empowered leaders. Many of them go to college and achieve dreams of becoming doctors and professionals. Gustavo Dudamel, a graduate of El Sistema, went on to become the conductor for the Los Angeles Philharmonic. The spirit of harmony learned by playing in a music ensemble creates a cultural pride, which transfers from symphony to life. The moving stories of these children are captured in the film *El Sistema*.

According to founder Abreu, music is a social right for all people. He says, "From the minute a child's taught to play a musical instrument, he is no longer poor."[4] Song lines are now extended from Latin America to the rest of the world, as El Sistema is being replicated in thirty other countries, including the United States.

Musical Diplomacy

Mahatma Gandhi once said, "If I had any influence, I should have great musicians attending every congress or conference and teaching mass music."[5]

Musical diplomacy is not a new idea. Long before I traveled to Iraq, historical song lines had been spread across the world, as the U.S. government recognized the power of music for cross-national relationship building. This may have served a political purpose, but at the same time it showed many performers just how far-reaching their sound could be.

In the post–World War II, Cold War era, the U.S. State Department sent Louis Armstrong to play throughout Africa, Europe, and Asia as a cultural ambassador. A long line of jazz artists, including Dave Brubeck, Max Roach, and Dizzy Gillespie, followed.

The horn was eventually passed to New Orleans trumpeter Wynton Marsalis, leader of the Lincoln Center Jazz Orchestra. In 2010, Marsalis and his group brought American jazz to street parades, performances, and clinics in Havana, Cuba. At a time when travel to Cuba was restricted for Americans, the trip created an extraordinary exchange, including the discovery of common African rhythms that underscore jazz and Cuban rumba alike. There is a message spoken in the freedom of improvisational jazz and the joy of connection; no translation needed. In an interview with *60 Minutes* correspondent Morley Safer, Marsalis said, "Through music we create community; we speak to the human soul."[6]

One day, by coincidence, I happened to catch a National Public Radio interview with jazz musician Chris Byars, who had just returned from a tour of the Middle East sponsored by Rhythm Road, a Jazz at Lincoln Center program. Since its inception in 1995, Rhythm Road has sent 150 musicians to more than one hundred countries. Chris had played in Iraq, and we started a dialogue via e-mail, sharing the feeling of playing music with and for "enemy" audiences. I shared that when I traveled to Iraq, I had never felt so at home in a place I'd been so afraid to visit. We both agreed that although we went to give, we received so much more. The reforming happened in us just as much as, or more than, in the places we traveled.

Orchestras of Change

Music's medicine is not only about change; it is also about exchange. Two of my favorite examples of orchestras that have created cultural exchange and traveled to places of political tension are the New York Philharmonic's trip to North Korea and the Iraqi National Symphony Orchestra performing in Washington, D.C.

In 2008, during a time of global tension over nuclear disarmament, the New York Philharmonic became the first-ever American orchestra to perform in North Korea. Their performance was broadcast on Korean television, reaching thousands of residents beyond the live audience members.

What moved me about the story was the magic that happened at the end of the concert. After the Americans played both countries' national anthems, they concluded with a well-loved Korean folk song. The Korean audience stood, waved, and applauded for three encores. American musicians waved back while wiping tears from their eyes. It was the first time many philharmonic members had been moved to tears on stage. The warm reception and the powerful statement of musical diplomacy touched both the North Korean audience and certainly the American musicians.

In 2003, the Iraqi National Symphony Orchestra came to Washington, D.C., for a performance with the U.S. National Symphony Orchestra. The concert featured cellist Yo-Yo Ma, a Culture Connect Ambassador of the Department of State. In a ripple of generosity, a private American organization raised funds to send the Iraqi symphony home with new instruments. Another group donated the musical scores of five hundred classical compositions. It didn't end the war in Iraq, but it reminds us that music brings out the best in us.

As I was writing this book, drinking tea at Starbucks, I noticed the quotation on my paper cup from "The Way I See It" series. It was from cellist Yo-Yo Ma:[7]

What I look for in musicians is generosity.
There is so much to learn from and about each other's culture.
Great creativity begins with tolerance.

Virtual Ensembles

In the neutral landscape of the digital universe, song lines are being woven through virtual bands and choirs that defy the physical distance between us. The result is a new model of collaboration, launching a vision and soundtrack of the world in harmony.

Inspired by a YouTube video clip of a young girl practicing her part for a choral piece that he had written, composer and conductor Eric Whitacre had a vision to create a virtual choir. He uploaded a video of himself conducting the score of *Lux Aurumque, Light and Gold,* his original composition. He invited open auditions by video clips. Instead of the nervous feeling of performing in front of judges, these submissions were shot in the homes and bedrooms of the singers, wearing their headphones to sing along with the tracks.

Whitacre's team then wove together 185 voices from twelve countries into a sublime video, which aired on YouTube and soon went viral, with more than two million views and growing. In small cubes strung together as if floating in the stars, the diverse singers are like a choir of angels laying song lines in the ethers of the virtual cosmos. The video brings tears, and the rich harmonies of the orchestration create goose bumps. We can sense the potential of world harmony.

Testimonials on YouTube show the healing responses both for choir members and audiences alike. Depressed viewers feel lifted, and choir members feel a sense of community with fellow singers they have never met. It seems the health benefits of ensemble membership may extend into digital ensembles as well. Whitacre describes himself as someone who dreamed of becoming a pop star. Instead, through his videos, he now conducts in the stars and is making stars of some amazing amateur singers. His next project, a Virtual Choir 2.0, took the original idea and made it bigger, including more than two thousand voices from fifty-eight countries. *Water Night,* his third effort, features 3,746 singers from seventy-three countries. Can you think of a better way to bring that many nations together in a peace talk?

Virtual bands are also using technology to defy borders. Inspired by the sound of street musicians in a New York subway station, Mark Johnson recorded street performances in more than ten countries, showing people singing along to "Stand by Me." Street musicians may be amateurs (which comes from the French word *amore,* which means "to love"), but these musicians play with passion and heart, even as they play for the "change" given by passers-by. Johnson's YouTube video went viral and launched the Playing for Change Foundation, which raises money for music schools in Africa and Nepal. The organization continues to create more videos; they also produce live music tours and hold an annual Playing for Change International Peace Day.

Sonic Revolution—In Real Time

Thanks to the Internet, musical service happens at the speed of a click. And the process of forwarding videos—or "word of mouse"—makes the music medicine go right where it's needed. It's like a "vein" to the world, a pathway through which music's medicine can proliferate the body of humanity.

To send our respect, love, and compassion to Japan after the 2011 earthquake and tsunami, a group of drummers at the Remo Recreational Music Center in North Hollywood and I made a video showing us playing the Japanese rhythm Taiko Matsuri. I posted it in my newsletter and sent it to my colleagues and friends in Japan. To see this video, search for it at youtube.com/ubdrumcircles. The Japanese people forwarded the video to their friends as well, and the responses were quite moving. I got great responses from complete strangers, thanking us for the rhythmic energy and the healing medicine of music.

When Haiti faced the earthquake that killed affected million people in 2010, a group of four facilitators and myself created a drum-circle benefit. Bonnie Devlin, a friend who had studied drumming in Haiti, created a YouTube clip of a traditional Haitian rhythm called *Ibo,* a folkloric beat from the Ibo people that represents liberation. *(Listen to track 2 in the orchestrating change playlist.)*

We sent out the video to the drum community so they could learn the beat. More than one hundred drummers came together at the World Beat Center in San Diego, all dressed in red, according to Haitian tradition. The drummers raised financial aid, and more importantly, they raised energy and prayers for the soul recovery, the inner structure of the people of Haiti. It wove the virtual with the physical, the prayer with the percussion, and created a digitally enhanced model of musical compassion.

The sheer outreach available through the Internet creates a new dimension of participation in orchestrating change. In this virtual peace rally, instead of fighting against something, music is singing in a new era.

Consider the math of this sonic revolutionary change. In the 1963 Civil Rights March on Washington, a quarter million people joined Martin Luther King Jr. to prevent racial discrimination. In 2003, between January and April, in thousands of events, an estimated thirty-six million people worldwide protested against the Iraq War. When you add up the cumulative number of hits on YouTube of just four music videos that orchestrate change—the virtual choir, "Stand by Me," U2's 2009 Rose Bowl Concert, and Farhad Darya in Afghanistan—you get a total of 41.2 million hits. That's 165 times the number of people at the March on Washington and greater than the entire world's protests against the Iraq War. Watching a video may not be the same as the action of marching on Washington, but I'd say we are ushering in a sonic revolution in the digital spheres, a revolution that can reach the homes of millions, no matter where we are.

Medicine for the Planet

Perhaps the greatest example of musical service to the world is reinvigorating the traditional uses of music medicine in resonance with the planet. Tribal people in many parts of the world sing to the waters, oceans, mountains, and forests. It's the law of harmony, giving back to that which feeds and sustains us.

Nature is affected by music just as we are. When classical or soothing music is played two to three hours a day, plants grow twice as large, bending as much as fifteen degrees toward the stereo.[8] As we know, live music amplifies the effect. Just imagine the power of singing or playing to nature; then imagine it further amplified by banding together with others in harmony.

First thing in the morning, my Lakota teachers rise and face the east to drum and chant a morning song. Music has long been a sacred offering to Mother Earth for First Nation's people. Sacred songs are sung to the stones, water, and fire. As we face the destruction of eco-harmony, which is making species extinct and causing damage to our forests and oceans, these practices are needed even more today.

When I traveled to the coast of Brazil, I got up in the mornings to walk along the ocean. I saw roses washing up at my feet in the morning tides. It's part of the Yoruba tradition to offer flowers to the ocean while singing to

Yemanja (the spirit of the ocean). The *orishas,* gods and goddesses, are made of nature's elements. The Brazilian Condomblé religion has songs, dances, flowers, and colors specific to each orisha. No matter what spiritual tradition or beliefs we hold, these rituals can honor our seas and waters. Nature is the ultimate interfaith temple. *(Listen to track 6 in the online orchestrating change playlist.)*

At the Honoring the Sea ceremony at the 2011 World Festival of Sacred Music in Santa Monica, California, I joined six hundred musicians from seven different cultural ensembles to support the local indigenous tribal people, the Tungva, in making offerings of rhythm and dance to the Pacific Ocean. I helped organize an international drum ensemble to perform and parade in the ceremony. People tossed flowers into the ocean, like at the ceremonies I'd attended in Brazil and Bali. We played rhythms for an entire afternoon, and then we stood in silence as the sun disappeared into the horizon, making its offering to the ocean as well. The day demonstrated how we can revive the ancient music medicine ways of offering music to nature.

Much like the feeling we have when a loved one is sick, witnessing nature's diseases can cause a feeling of helplessness. Music gives us a tool to contribute. After a wildfire near my home in Southern California, my teacher Kathy Hull and I went to a beautiful oak grove, where amazingly the trees had survived the devastation. Standing in ashes on the charred earth, we sang and drummed for the new growth that we knew was coming in nature's remarkable ecological rhythm of death and rebirth. The experience taught me to listen more deeply to the earth's song requests and to answer the call.

Final Chorus

Listen and you will hear the voices of performers becoming reformers as change is breaking out globally through the unity of music. The soundtrack is already playing. Freedom songs accompany social movements that call for change and a better, more harmonious treatment of one another. Music's medicine offers its resonance to the people and the planet in this time of transformation.

GUIDED PRACTICES FOR ORCHESTRATING CHANGE

In giving our music, we expand ourselves and connect to a greater purpose. As we conclude our journey through all the elements of music's medicine, here are some practices for conscious listening and music making for orchestrating change. Consider these practices as ways of contributing to the ocean of sound that encircles the planet and connects you to the song lines around the world.

Guided Practices for Conscious Listening

Listening to the World's Songs
(All tracks from the online orchestrating change playlist)
Conscious listening to the sounds of world music attunes your ears to new languages, rhythms, scales, harmonies, and the use of silence. Music defines cultures. Through conscious listening with an open heart, you travel to other lands without a passport. It does require openness, because some of this music might sound foreign to you.

I've created a playlist filled with the four elements of music's medicine: Haitian and Afro-Brazilian rhythms, Hebrew chanting melodies, rich harmonies of an Afro-Gypsy guitar ensemble and a Mediterranean orchestra, and the peaceful quiet of Zimbabwean healing music.

Listen beyond the words and tune into the intent of the music. Can you feel its meaning? Let the music expand your soul and fall into the rhythm, melody, harmony, and silence of the world.

Be the Change
It is the action call of His Holiness the Dalai Lama to create peace through more music festivals. Find a local cultural music event that is new to your ears. Travel outside your comfort zone and go on a sonic expedition. The movement outside our comfort zone is often a catalyst for personal growth and transformation. It may just be a concert or live music at an ethnic restaurant. I like to hear live ethnic music in the same way people like to go out for ethnic food—it feeds me. Search YouTube for a music video from a

culture you've always been interested in. Start with the ethnic food you love, and listen to the music that defines that culture.

Here are tips I've developed over the years for attending a cultural music event. Always carry small gifts for those who assist you or who deserve honoring. It may be the performers, volunteers, or cooks. Get to know the people. Be curious. Your interest in other cultures is often the highest compliment and will be received with gratitude. Listen to the music with an open mind, and notice the differences and commonalities in the rhythm, melody, harmony, or silence. And most of all, participate. Dance or sing along when invited, and enjoy the food that matches the music. Be the change by bridging cultures through music.

Guided Practices for Expressing

Singing to the Earth

(Track 6)

What is your favorite aspect of nature? What moves you most deeply? Is it trees, flowers, ocean, rivers, wind, or mountains? Notice what time of day your favorite element is most prevalent. Is it the birds in the morning or the humming of crickets at night, the sunshine that breaks through the dark of night or the sun as it sets? If there has been damage done to the nature around you, how can you make a music offering to its healing?

Select one of nature's elements to honor through music. Honor nature in your own act of musical service today. Ideally, you can go on a hike or walk and take a moment to offer your music. You can use a song or just a drumbeat. Tribal people sing traditional songs to nature, and you may already know these songs or have access to learn them. There may be a nature song you learned as a child at summer camp. I still remember singing, "I love the mountains, I love the rolling hills, I love the flowers, I love the daffodils, boom de a da, boom de a da." Your nature song might even be a lyric of a Beatles song, like "Here comes the sun." So much music is inspired by nature that it's easy to find something that will resonate. If not, you may have to make up your own or create a wordless chant that you can offer outside in nature to your favorite element. Sometimes if you listen very carefully, nature will teach you its song.

When you are finished, pause and listen. What do you hear? Are there more birds singing, crickets sounding, and wind blowing? How does nature respond to your call?

Random Acts of Music

Like random acts of kindness, the magic of music medicine can happen in spontaneous and unexpected ways. I carry a small Native American flute in my purse or hiking bag and a small drum in my car for those random moments when a sonic contribution just feels right.

Once I was delayed in an airport because of bad weather. I happened to have my African djembe drum with me. As the customer service agents were experiencing the stress of angry travelers lined up at the ticket counter, I sat and softly began to play my drum. People started tapping their feet; some were smiling. The flight coordinator motioned me to the desk and held the loud speaker over my drum. The good vibrations were suddenly heard throughout the terminal. It created an eruption of laughter, surprise, and applause at the end. That random act of musical service transformed the energy of the terminal from tension to percussion. When you find yourself in a situation that needs transforming, it's good to have music.

When you find yourself in a situation that could use an energy change, consider toning in the space, singing, chanting, or using an instrument to create a new vibration. Think of what you need in order to prepare yourself to be ready for a random act of music. Consider getting a small drum or flute to fit in your hiking pack. Moments of magic in music can happen spontaneously. You cannot plan them. But you can be ready.

Becoming a Reformer

Musical service is in your hands. You hold the conductor's baton. This book has offered you many tools for your own musical healing and has also suggested ways to extend the inner music of your spirit into the outer music of the world. If you desire to give back from the great reservoir of creativity, there are ways beyond my suggestions to use digital forces to make a great sonic contribution.

Are you inspired to lead? If so, you may want to create a chanting circle, become trained in facilitating a drum circle, form a sound-healing group, or even form a band. Are you inspired to create sound as an offering to friends in need of healing? Is there a way you can weave more music into your work, bringing specifically selected music into the teacher's lounge or some other creative way to infuse music's medicine into the daily rhythms of work?

How has music transformed you? How can you share the gift of music with the world in your own unique way? Just asking that question will create a call-and-response with your own inner truth. Musical service is an expression of the inner music that is activated in you. Giving it away only amplifies that unlimited creative well within you. An answer is waiting.

ANNOTATED PLAYLIST FOR ORCHESTRATING CHANGE

To stream this music, visit SoundsTrue.com/MusicMedicine.

1. "Oseh Shalom," YofiYah, *Kabalah Kirtan*
The playlist opens with a devotional call to peace. *Oseh* means "He who makes," and *shalom* means "peace." Listen to the end of the recording, as the music slows into a deep, resonant chorus of shalom, sung in a single chord of harmony.

2. "Ibo," Geoff Johns, *Bakongo!*
In traditional rhythm cultures, rhythm is inseparable from dance and chant in ceremony and ritual. This Haitian rhythm is dedicated to celebrating freedom. The dance that accompanies it involves the motions of breaking free from chains. As the recording progresses, the beat changes, rising to a new rhythm of freedom and celebration.

3. "Del Meeravad Ze Dastam," Dastan Ensemble with Shahram Nazeri, *Through Eternity*
This rich Persian music presents a very different tonality. Hear the heart of the world, singing the phrase that means "my heart is slipping from my grasp."

4. "Ker Kerane," Shaman's Dream, *African Dream*
The lyrics of Senegalese Sufi holy man Cheick Alhmadou Bamba translate as, "In the morning or in darkness, there is always light." A synthesis of global sounds highlights the accompanying music, which includes Moroccan bongos, African djembe, Nigerian talking drum, and keyboards.

5. "Candombe del Mono Azul," Pepe Danza, *Drum Prayers*
Listen to the waves becoming rhythm and song. Dance to this original composition based on Uruguay's national rhythm, Candombe. Using conga, samba bells, ocean sounds, and chant, Pepe Danza brings his own heritage to life with traditional call-and-response chorus chanting.

6. "Yemaja for Two," Silvia Nakkach, *Medicine Melodies*
Yemaja is the *orisha* of the ocean waters in the Afro-Brazilian orisha tradition.
This beautiful traditional chant is sung to the ocean all over Brazil. Enjoy
Silvia Nakkach's enchanting voice. She leads sound-healing trips to Brazil
through her Vox Mundi school.

7. "Mira," Priyo, *Gypsy Moon*
Enjoy the Afro-Gypsy blend in Priyo's guitar playing, which bridges flamenco
with African beats.

8. "Shumba YaNgwasha," Erica Azim, *Mbira Dreams World*
In the tradition of Shona music from Zimbabwe, Erica Azim, the first
non-Zimbabwean to learn Shona music, creates a soft, meditative composition. The *mbira* (pronounced "m-bee-ra") is a thumb piano, in which metal
keys are attached to a wooden board and fitted inside a gourd as a resonator.
Shumba YaNgwasha means "voice of the ancestors."

Postlude

Through this journey, we have traced the ancient roots of the healing properties of music's medicine. In each musical element, we have considered the scientific evidence and spiritual traditions that underscore the impact of bringing each of the four aspects of music's medicine into your lifestyle for healing, health, well-being, and personal growth. The result is a discovery of all the elements that are within you in the fifth element of the inner music.

Side Effects

As you work with the medicine of this book, you may notice some changes in yourself and in your life. Much of life may sound different to you as you move from loving music to living music. Like any medicine, music does have side effects, but they are good ones.

You may become "rhythmatized." You may hear the rhythm of brushing your teeth at night and start to tap along with the groove. You may find yourself sitting at a traffic light, rocking out to the beat of the turning signal, never noticing that the light has changed to green. You may hear the groove in the fan spinning above your head when you go to sleep at night.

You may become "melodified." You may notice the melodies of birds singing in the morning. You may hear the music in spoken voices in conversations. You may detect undercurrents of emotions or even a lack of feeling in the monotone speech of a friend. You may hear a great resonance coming through your own voice as you allow yourself to sing more freely in those secret rehearsal rooms of the shower or the car. You may detect truth and wisdom in the tonality of the words of a beloved teacher. Your heart may be moved by songs in deeper ways. You will hear differently and more deeply.

You may become "harmonized." You may feel a greater sense of connection to the sonic presence in all things. You may notice a greater ability to blend with others in projects, or you may tune in to the times when a conductor is needed and you lift your baton. You may notice you are better at recognizing when to take the lead and when to support, when to be the stronger voice or the harmonizing sound. You may find yourself lingering in nature when you hear the harmony of the elements in their endless symphony; no concert tickets required. You become part of the law of harmony, more aware of the balance of giving and receiving, tuning yourself to greater levels of beauty and collaboration.

You may become "restified." You may become more aware of silence and linger in its song. You may become more comfortable with periods of pause and silence. You may feel less anxiety in the quiet moments of mystery's breath. You may discover the love of silent retreat time and notice how it births more creativity in your life.

And lastly, you may become "sonified." You may experience a greater resonance of your inner music and a desire to express your song. You may catch yourself tapping, humming, whistling, moving in an expression of your inner musical spirit. It happens naturally, without thinking. You may notice you have let go of some of the barriers to your own creativity. You may catch yourself making up songs, remembering the musical freedom of childhood and nurturing the seeds of creative musical expression within yourself. You may notice the positive effect of your own resonance on others in your life, sharing your musical spirit freely and with an open heart. This is a good thing, for you have awakened all the elements of music within you, becoming an instrument of groove, song, harmony, and silence on the planet.

Lasting Effects

Music never dies. It has been with us since the beginning, and it extends into eternity. Sound reverberates, and so do the benefits of music in our lives. I leave you with this blessing of the four elements of music:

May your body dance in the rhythm of life.

May your heart sing a melody of love.

May your soul harmonize with all of creation.

May your mind rest in the silence of peace.

Notes

Chapter 1. Sound Check

1. George Leonard, *The Silent Pulse* (Salt Lake City, UT: Gibbs Smith, 2006), 14.
2. National Association of Music Merchants, "2006 Music USA: NAMM Global Report," accessed May 6, 2011, wannaplaymusic.com/gallup_poll.
3. National Association of Music Merchants, "2009 Public Attitudes Toward Music," Gallup Poll accessed May 6, 2011. Used with permission.
4. Norwich Union, "UK: Norwich Union Reveals the Nation's Top Regrets," July 17, 2007, accessed August 6, 2011, aviva.co.uk/media-centre/ story/3392/norwich-union-reveals-the-nations-top-regrets/.
5. Christine Stevens, "The UpBeat Philosophy: You Are Musical!" *UpBeat Drum Circles,* 2005, ubdrumcircles.com/article_musical.html.
6. Barry Bittman et al., "Recreational Music-Making Modulates the Human Stress Response: A Preliminary Individualized Gene Expression Strategy," *Medical Science Monitor* 11 (2005): 31–40.

Chapter 2. The Medicine of Music

1. Mark Fox, "E-commerce Business Models for the Music Industry," *Popular Music and Society* 27, no. 2 (2004): 201.
2. Pamela Tsai, "Interview with Yo-Yo Ma: A Personal Journey on a Cultural Silk Road," *The Epoch Times,* August 16, 2010, accessed November 26, 2011, theepochtimes.com/n2/arts-entertainment/an-interview-with-yo-yo-ma-silk-road-chinese-music-41028.html.
3. Sheldon Cohen, Denise Janicki-Deverts, and Gregory E. Miller, "Psychological Stress and Disease," *Journal of the American Medical Association* 298, no. 14 (2007): 1685–87.
4. Pat Love, *The Truth about Love: The Highs, the Lows, and How You Can Make It Last Forever* (New York: Simon & Schuster, 2001), 171–72.
5. Hazrat Inayat Khan, *The Music of Life: The Inner Nature and Effects of Sound* (New Lebanon, NY: Omega Publications, 2005), 63.

6. Joshua M. Greene, *Here Comes the Sun: The Spiritual and Musical Journey of George Harrison* (Hoboken, NJ: John Wiley and Sons, 2006), 210.

7. Pete S. Catches, Sr., and Peter V. Catches, eds. *Sacred Fireplace (Oceti Wakan): Life and Teachings of a Lakota Medicine Man* (Santa Fe, NM: Clear Light Publications, 1999), 181.

8. John Neihardt, *Black Elk Speaks: Being the Life Story of a Holy Man of the Oglala Sioux as told through John G. Neihardt* (Lincoln, NE: University of Nebraska Press, 1961), 199.

9. Lorin Roche, *The Radiance Sutras: 112 Tantra Yoga Teachings for Opening to the Divine in Everyday Life* (Marina del Rey, CA: Syzygy Creations, 2008), sutras 16, 60.

10. Laura A. Mitchell and Raymond A. R. MacDonald, "An Experimental Investigation of the Effects of Preferred and Relaxing Music Listening on Pain Perception," *Journal of Music Therapy* 43 (2006): 295–316.

11. Avram Goldstein, "Thrills in Response to Music and Other Stimuli," *Physiological Psychology* 8, no. 1 (1980): 126–29.

12. Barry B. Bittman et al., "Composite Effects of Group Drumming Music Therapy on Modulation of Neuroendocrine-Immune Parameters in Normal Subjects," *Journal of Alternative Therapy* January 2001: 38–47.

13. Gunter Kreutz et al., "Effects of Choir Singing or Listening on Secretory Immunoglobulin A, Cortisol, and Emotional State," *Journal of Behavioral Medicine* 27 (2004): 623–35.

Chapter 3. Rhythm: Medicine for the Body

1. Samuel Beckett, *Waiting for Godot: A Tragicomedy in Two Acts* (New York: Grove Press, 1982), 41.

2. Véronique L. Roger et al., "Heart Association Heart Disease and Stroke Statistics 2011 Update: A Report from the American Heart Association," *Circulation* 123 (2011): e18–e209.

3. Ibid.

4. Ibid.

5. Michael Thaut, *Rhythm, Music, and the Brain: Scientific Foundations and Clinical Applications (Studies on New Music Research)* (New York: Routledge, Taylor & Francis Group, 2005).

6. Gerald C. McIntosh et al., "Rhythmic Auditory-Motor Facilitation of Gait Patterns in Patients with Parkinson's Disease," *Journal of Neurology Neurosurgery and Psychiatry* 62 (1997): 22–26.

7. Alicia Clair, Barry Bernstein, and Gary Johnson, "Rhythm Playing Characteristics in Persons with Severe Dementia, Including Those with Probable Alzheimer's Type," *Journal of Music Therapy* 32 (1995): 113–31.

8. Barry B. Bittman et al., "Drumming Strengthens Immune System: Composite Effects of Group Drumming Music Therapy on Modulation of Neuroendocrine-Immune Parameters in Normal Subjects," *Journal of Alternative Therapy* 7 (2001): 38–47.

9. Masatada Wachi et al., "Recreational Music-Making Modulates Natural Killer Cell Activity, Cytokines, and Mood States in Corporate Employees," *Medical Science Monitor* 13 (2007): 57–70.

10. Barry B. Bittman et al., "Recreational Music-Making: A Cost-Effective Group Interdisciplinary Strategy for Reducing Burnout and Improving Mood States in Long-Term Care Workers," *Advances in Mind-Body Medicine* 19, no. 3/4 (2003): 4–15.

11. Barry B. Bittman, Larry Dickson, and Kim Coddington, "Creative Musical Expression as a Catalyst for Quality of Life Improvement in Inner-City Adolescents Placed in a Court-Referred Residential Treatment Program," *Advances in Mind-Body Medicine* 24, no. 1 (2009): 8–19.

12. Barry B. Bittman et al., "Recreational Music-Making (RMM) Inspires Creativity and Bonding in Long-Term Care Residents," *Provider* (2003/2004): 39–41.

13. Barry B. Bittman et al., "Recreational Music-Making: An Integrative Group Intervention for Reducing Burnout and Improving Mood States in First Year Associate Degree Nursing Students: Insights and Economic Impact," *International Journal of Nursing Education and Scholarship* 1 (2004).

14. Costas Karageorghis, Leighton Jones, and D. P. Stuart, "Psychological Effects of Music Tempi During Exercise," *International Journal of Sports Medicine* 29 (2008): 613–19.

15. Costas Karageorghis et al., "Psychophysical and Ergogenic Effects of Synchronous Music During Treadmill Walking," *Journal of Sport and Exercise Psychology* 31 (2009): 18–36.

16. Mabry Doyle, "Cultivating Indigenous World Awareness," *Awareness* (July–August 2000).

17. Babatunde Olatunji, "Dance to the Beat of My Drum," *Drums of Passion: The Beat* (Portland, OR: Blue Heron Records), BLU 706, track 1.

18. Mickey Hart and Fredric Lieberman, *Spirit into Sound: The Magic of Music* (Petaluma, CA: Acid Test Productions, 1999), 145.

19. Heidi Varian, *The Way of Taiko* (Berkeley, CA: Stone Bridge Press, 2005), 17.

20. Layne Redmond, *Invoking the Muse* (Boulder, CO: Sounds True, 2004).

21. Layne Redmond, *When the Drummers Were Women: A Spiritual History of Rhythm* (New York: Three Rivers Press, 1997).

22. Joseph Epes Brown, ed., *The Sacred Pipe: Black Elk's Account of the Seven Rites of the Oglala Sioux* (Norman: University of Oklahoma Press, 1953, 1989), 26.

23. Arthur Hull, "How to Facilitate Drum Circles" (presentation at the Hawaii Facilitators Playshop, Oahu, Hawaii, August 8–15, 2000).

24. Allessandra Belloni, *Rhythm Is the Cure* (Pacific, MO: Mel Bay, 2007).

25. Sue Woodman, "A Healthy Beat," *AARP My Generation,* November–December 2002, 14.

Chapter 4. Melody: Medicine for the Heart

1. Hazrat Inayat Khan, *The Music of Life: The Inner Nature and Effects of Sound* (New Lebanon, NY: Omega Publications, 2005), 128.

2. University of Leicester, "University of Leicester Produces the First Ever World Map of Happiness: Happiness Is . . . Being Healthy, Wealthy, and Wise," (press release, August 1, 2006).

3. Editors, "The State of Our Unions," *Psychology Today,* January/February (2000): 10.

4. Jennifer Baker, "Divorce Rate in America," DivorceRate, accessed August 23, 2011, divorcerate.org.

5. Véronique L. Roger et al., "Heart Disease and Stroke Statistics 2011 Update: A Report from the American Heart Association," *Circulation* 123 (2011): 18–201.

6. Philip Beaman and Tim Williams, "Earworms 'Stuck Song Syndrome': Towards a Natural History of Intrusive Thoughts," *British Journal of Psychology* 101: 637–53.

7. Peter G. Hepper, "An Examination of Fetal Learning Before and After Birth," *The Irish Journal of Psychology* 12 (1991): 95–107.

8. Judy Platinga and Laurel J. Trainor, "Memory for Melody: Infants Use a Relative Pitch Code," *Cognition* 98 (2005): 1–11.

9. Sandra E. Trehub, Dale Bull, and Leigh A. Thorpe, "Infants' Perception of Melodies: The Role of Melodic Contour," *Child Development* 55 (1984): 821–30.

10. Peter Ostwald, "Musical Behavior in Early Childhood," *Developmental Medicine and Child Neurology* 15 (1973): 367–75.

11. David J. Hole et al., "Impaired Lung Function and Mortality Risk in Men and Women: Findings from the Renfrew and Paisley Prospective Population Study," *British Medical Journal* 313 (1996): 711–15.

12. Robert J. Hancox et al., "Systematic Inflammation and Lung Function in Young Adults," *Thorax* 62 (2007): 1064–68.

13. Gunter Kreutz et al., "Effects of Choir Singing or Listening on Secretory Immunoglobulin A, Cortisol, and Emotional State," *Journal of Behavioral Medicine* 27 (2004): 623–35.

14. Kathleen McCormick, "A Heartfelt High C Workout," *American Journal of Nursing* 86 (1986): 993.

15. Ana Mendes et al., "Effects of Vocal Training on Respiratory Kinematics during Singing Tasks," *Folia Phoniatrica et Logopaedica* 58, no. 5 (2006): 363–77.

16. A. B. Birnbaum, "The Song in the Courts of the Tzadikim in Poland," *Haolam* (1908).

17. Ruth Beebe Hill, *Hanta Yo: An American Saga* (New York: Doubleday, 1979), 28.

18. David Steindl-Rast, with Sharon Lebell, *The Music of Silence: A Sacred Journey through the Hours of the Days* (Berkeley, CA: Ulysses Press, 1998), 16.

19. Paramahansa Yogananda, *Cosmic Chants* (Los Angeles: Self-Realization Fellowship, 1996), 29.

20. Nicholas J. Conard, Maria Malina, and Susanne C. Münzel, "New Flutes Document the Earliest Musical Tradition in Southwestern Germany," *Nature* 460 (2009): 737–40.

21. Katie Moisse, "Music Therapy Helps Gabrielle Giffords Find Her Voice after Tucson Shooting," *ABC News,* March 8, 2011.

22. Angeles Arrien, *The Four-Fold Way: Walking the Paths of the Warrior, Teacher, Healer, and Visionary* (San Francisco: Harper, 1993), 85.

23. Mattie J. T. Stepanek, *Journey through Heartsongs* (New York: Hyperion, 2001), 3.

24. Jonathan Goldman, *Vocal Toning the Chakras.* (Boulder, CO: Sounds True), 18.

Chapter 5. Harmony: Medicine for the Soul

1. Rabindranath Tagore, *The Fugitive* (London: MacMillan Press, 1921), 19.

2. William Wray, *Leonardo da Vinci in His Own Words* (London: Arcturus Press, 2005), 166.

3. U.S. Department of Justice, "National Crime Victimization Survey, Criminal Victimization 2007," Bureau of Justice Statistics Bulletin (Washington, D.C.: U.S. Department of Justice, 2008).

4. Child Help, "National Child Abuse Statistics: Child Abuse in America," accessed August 28, 2011, childhelp.org/pages/statistics.

5. U.S. Department of Veterans Affairs, *Review of State Variances in VA Disability Compensation Payments,* report no. 05-00765-137 (Washington, D.C.: VA Office of Inspector General, 2005), accessed November 29, 2011, veteransnewsroom.com/files/press/VETERANS-Fact-Sheet-Veterans.pdf.

6. John Cacioppo, James Fowler, and Nicholas Christakis, "Alone in the Crowd: The Structure and Spread of Loneliness in a Large Social Network," *Journal of Personality and Social Psychology* 97 (2009): 977–91.

7. Judy Foreman, "Loneliness Can Be the Death of the U.S.," *Boston Globe,* April 22, 1996.

8. Joshua Leeds, *The Power of Sound* (Rochester, VT: Healing Arts Press, 2010).

9. Vittorio Gallese, "A Unifying View of the Basis of Social Cognition," *Trends in Cognitive Sciences* 8 (2004): 396–402.

10. Christian Keysers et al., "Audiovisual Mirror Neurons and Action Recognition," *Experimental Brain Research* 153 (2003): 628–36.

11. Evelyn Kohler et al., "Hearing Sounds, Understanding Actions: Action Representation in Mirror Neurons," *Science* 297 (2002): 846–48.

12. Istvan Molnar-Szakacs and Katie Overy, "Being Together in Time: Musical Experience and the Mirror Neuron System," *Music Perception* (2009): 489–504.

13. Istvan Molnar-Szakacs and Katie Overy, "Music and Mirror Neurons: From Motion to 'E'motion," *Social Cognitive Affective Neuroscience* 1 (2006): 235–41.

14. Robert D. Putnam, *Bowling Alone: The Collapse and Revival of American Community* (New York: Simon & Schuster, 2000).

15. Chorus Impact Study, "How Children, Adults, and Communities Benefit from Choruses," Chorus America, 2009, accessed August 29, 2011, chorusamerica.org/about_choralsinging.cfm.

16. Stephen Clift and Grenville Hancox, "The Significance of Choral Singing for Sustaining Psychological Wellbeing: Findings from a Survey of Choristers in England, Australia, and Germany," *Music Performance Research* 3 (2010): 79–96.

17. Don Coffman and Mary Adamek, "The Contributions of Wind Band Participation to Quality of Life of Senior Adults," *Music Therapy Perspectives* 17 (1999): 27–31.

18. Robert J. Beck et al., "Choral Singing, Performance Perception, and Immune System Changes in Salivary Immunoglobulin A and Cortisol," *Music Perception* 18 (2000): 87–106.

19. Don Coffman and Mary Adamek, "The Contributions of Wind Band Participation to Quality of Life of Senior Adults," *Music Therapy Perspectives* 17 (1999): 27–31.

20. Dalai Lama, "Address to the World Festival of Sacred Music," speech presented at the World Festival of Sacred Music, Los Angeles, October 9, 1999.

21. Matthew 18:20 (New International Version).

22. Jean-Yves Leloup, *The Gospel of Mary Magdalene* (Rochester, VT: Inner Traditions, 2002), 63–64.

23. George R. Parulski, *A Path to Oriental Wisdom: Introductory Studies in Eastern Philosophy* (Burbank, CA: Ohara Publications, 1976).

Chapter 6. Silence: Medicine for the Mind

1. Jill Purce, "The Healing Voice" (lecture, Third International Sound Healing Conference, Santa Fe, NM, November 15, 2008).

2. George Michelson Foy, *Zero Decibels: The Quest for Absolute Silence* (New York: Scribner, 2010), 6.

3. Birgitta Berglund and Thomas Lindvall, eds., *Community Noise, Archives of the Centre for Sensory Research* 2, no. 1 (1995): 1–195.

4. George Michelson Foy, *Zero Decibels: The Quest for Absolute Silence* (New York: Scribner, 2010), 13.

5. Birgitta Berglund and Thomas Lindvall, eds., *Community Noise: Archives of the Centre for Sensory Research* 2, no. 1 (1995): 1–195.

6. Don Campbell and Alex Doman, *Healing at the Speed of Sound* (New York: Hudson Street Press, 2011).

7. Marilyn Elias, "'Mindful' Meditation Being Used in Hospitals and Schools," *USA Today,* June 8, 2009.

8. Paul McCartney, receiving the Library of Congress Gershwin Prize for Popular Song, June 2, 2010.

9. David Steindl-Rast and Sharon Lebell, *Music of Silence: A Sacred Journey through the Hours of the Day* (Berkeley, CA: Ulysses Press, 2001), 115.

10. John Cage, *Silence, Lectures, and Writings by John Cage* (Middletown, CT: Wesleyan University Press, 1961), 7.

11. Luciano Bernardi, Cesare Porta, and Peter Sleight, "Cardiovascular, Cerebrovascular, and Respiratory Changes Induced by Different Types of Music in Musicians and Non-Musicians: The Importance of Silence," *Heart* 92 (2006): 445–52.

12. Steve Silberman, "Placebos Are Getting More Effective: Drugmakers Are Desperate to Know Why," *Wired,* 17 (2009).

13. Ted J. Kaptchuk et al, "Placebos without Deception: A Randomized Controlled Trial in Irritable Bowel Syndrome," *PLoS ONE,* 5, no. 12 (2010).

14. Rients Ritskes et al., "MRI Scanning during Zen Meditation: The Picture of Enlightenment," *Constructivism in the Human Sciences* 8 (2003): 85–89.

15. Sara Lazar et al., "Functional Brain Mapping of the Relaxation Response and Meditation," *Autonomic Nervous System, Neuroreport* 11 (2000): 1581–85.

16. Erik Ryding, Björn Brådvik, and David H. Ingvar, "Silent Speech Activates Prefrontal Cortical Regions Asymmetrically, as Well as Speech-Related Areas in the Dominant Hemisphere," *Brain and Language* 52 (1996): 435–51.

17. Richard J. Davidson et al., "Alterations in Brain and Immune Function Produced by Mindfulness Meditation," *Psychosomatic Medicine* 65 (2003): 564–70.

18. Ibid.
19. Sri Chinmoy, *The Source of Music: Music and Mantra for Self-Realization* (New York: Aum Publications, 1999), 4.
20. Paramahansa Yogananda, *Cosmic Chants: Spiritualized Songs for Divine Communion,* 6th ed. (Los Angeles: Self-Realization Fellowship, 1996), 43.
21. David Steindl-Rast and Sharon Lebell, *Music of Silence: A Sacred Journey through the Hours of the Day* (Berkeley, CA: Ulysses Press, 2001), 104.
22. Annual Sleep in America, "Poll Exploring Connections with Communications Technology Use and Sleep" (press release, National Sleep Foundation, March 7, 2011).
23. Michael J. Breus, "Sleep Habits: More Important Than You Think," *WebMD,* 2004, webmd.com/sleep-disorders/guide/important-sleep-habits.

Chapter 7. Inner Music: Medicine for the Spirit

1. La Clochette, v12, Dec. 1912, 285.
2. Oscar Wilde, *The Picture of Dorian Gray and Other Writings* (New York: Random House, 1982), 204.
3. Mickey Hart and Frederick Lieberman, *Spirit into Sound: The Magic of Music* (Petaluma, CA: Acid Test Productions, 1999), 117.
4. Jonathan H. Ellerby, *Inspiration Deficit Disorder: The No-Pill Prescription to End High Stress, Low Energy, and Bad Habits* (Carlsbad, CA: Hay House, 2010), 93–98.
5. Janice Lloyd, "Antidepressant Use Skyrockets 400% in Two Decades," *USA Today,* October 19, 2011.
6. *Webster's New College Dictionary* 3rd ed., s.v. "music."
7. Jamie C. Kassler, *Inner Music: Hobbes, Hooke, and North on Internal Character* (London: Athlone Press, 1995), 198.
8. *Webster's New College Dictionary* 3rd ed., s.v. "resonance."
9. Charles J. Limb and Allen R. Braun, "Neural Substrates of Spontaneous Musical Performance: An fMRI Study of Jazz Improvisation," *PLoS ONE,* 3, no. 2 (2008).
10. Kenneth S. Aigen, "Popular Musical Styles in Nordoff-Robbins Clinical Improvisation," *Music Therapy Perspectives* 19 (2001): 31–44.
11. Wendy L. Magee, "A Comparison between the Use of Songs and Improvisation in Music Therapy with Adults Living with Acquired and Chronic Illness," *Australian Journal of Music Therapy* 18 (2007): 20.

12. Felicity Baker et al., "Therapeutic Songwriting in Music Therapy," *Nordic Journal of Music Therapy* 17, no. 2 (2008): 105–123.

13. Lorin Roche, "Ohm," Sanskrit Glossary, accessed October 23, 2011, lorinroche.com/Sanskrit-ar/sanskrit/om.html.

14. Daryai Lal Kapur, *Call of the Great Master* (New Delhi: Anupam Art Printers, 1964), 156.

15. Lorin Roche, *The Radiance Sutras: 112 Tantra Yoga Teachings for Opening to the Divine in Everyday Life* (Marina del Rey, CA: Syzygy Creations, 2008), sutra 91.

16. Ibid.

17. Coleman Barks, *The Essential Rumi—Each Note* (New York: Harper Collins, 1995), 103.

18. Lorin Roche, "Tantri," Sanskrit Glossary, accessed October 23, 2011, lorinroche.com/sanskrit-t/sanskrit-t/tantri.html.

19. Christine Stevens, "Reclaiming the Rhythm: An Interview with Rick Allen," *Percussive Notes* 40, no. 4 (2002): 54, 56.

Chapter 8. Orchestrating Change: Medicine for the World

1. Rick Rays, director, *Ten Questions for the Dalai Lama* (Monterey, CA: Monterey Media, 2006), DVD.

2. Christine Stevens, "One Inspired Rhythm in Iraq," *Making Music,* July 9, 2004.

3. Group participants of Kurdistan Save the Children Youth Activity Center, in discussion with the author, November 2007, Sulaimaniya, Iraq.

4. "José Abreu on Kids Transformed by Music" (video), TED: Ideas Worth Spreading. Filmed February 2009, ted.com/talks/jose_abreu_on_kids_transformed_by_music.html.

5. Richard Attenborough, *The Words of Gandhi* (New York: New Market Press, 1982), 58.

6. "Wynton Marsalis: America's Musical Ambassador," *60 Minutes,* December 26, 2010, by CBS; produced by David Browning and Diane Beasley; edited by Matt Danowski.

7. Yo-Yo Ma, "The Way I See It," #7. Starbucks coffee cup.

8. Don Robertson, "About Positive Music," accessed January 17, 2012, dovesong.com/positive_music/plant_experiments.asp.

Guide to Using Music Medicine for Personal and Professional Development

This resource guide offers tools and tips for incorporating music and sound into your work. It is organized by profession and purpose. Many of the guided practices are curriculum builders, tools for coaching and therapy, and creative ways to bring healing into your life.

There are forty-eight guided practices that follow the six key chapters of the book. By using these conscious listening and expressing practices, you can offer your students, clients, colleagues, and friends a healing experience with music that can be life changing. What follows are some ways to bring the drum medicine, song medicine, ensemble medicine, resting medicine, and resonance of music's medicine into your work.

Music Medicine for Self-Care

Music medicine begins with you, as a tool for self-care, stress reduction, healing, and life enhancement. Whether you desire to teach, coach, or treat clients and students with the tools presented in this book, it's best to begin with yourself. Now that we have travelled through the elements of music and their healing properties, here are tips for putting music's medicine into your life:

1. Determine what healing you want to create in your life. Are you looking to create more wellness, or do you want to heal your body, mind, spirit, heart, or soul? Are you interested in greater spirituality and better balance, or are you seeking a preventive health strategy? If you are a musician or artist, are you coming up against creative blocks or feeling a deeper source of your artistic expression wanting to come through you?

2. Assess yourself. Consider where you are in balance or off balance. What are your strengths and weaknesses? What are your places of greatest development, and what areas have been stifled or neglected? Do you need more rest? Do you need to feel freer in your body, to awaken your heart song, or to find

greater harmony with nature?

Sound assessment. In which element do you most thrive: rhythm, melody, harmony, silence, or inner music? In which element are you most deficient? If you are a musician, what aspect of music do you need to explore more?

Wellness assessment. Where do you need healing: in your body, mind, spirit, heart, or soul? In which do you feel strongest? How is your overall balance? What part of you is yearning for greater expression?

3. To create your individual music-medicine practice, choose guided practices in the areas where you want to strengthen yourself. If you already have a spiritual practice, how can you weave music into your current routine? At what time of day do you need support? Time of day is important; I often recommend that people choose a listening and expressing practice for the morning and evening, to bookend the day in the resonance of music's medicine.

Following are a few of the most popular techniques that can be easily woven into your routine or that can create a new foundation of music medicine in your life. They are organized by conscious listening and expressing, as well as by the type of medicine they bring.

Listening

Resting medicine: "Sound Savasana," in chapter 6 (page 123)

Drum medicine: "Drum Massage," in chapter 3 (page 46)

Song medicine: "Finding Your Power Song," in chapter 4 (page 74)

Ensemble medicine: "Soul Music Sharing," in chapter 5 (page 102)

Expressing

Song medicine: "Awaken Your Voice," in chapter 4 (page 75)

Drum medicine: "Heartbeat," in chapter 3 (page 48)

Resonance: "Morning Attunement," in chapter 7 (page 149)

Orchestrating change: "Singing to the Earth," in chapter 8 (page 170)

Music Medicine for Book Club Leaders

Questions for Discussion

1. In chapter 2, the author describes her work using drumming in Iraq for healing and peacemaking. Do you think this method would be helpful in other parts of the world?

2. In chapter 3, the author offers research on the scientific foundation of music for healing. Can you identify with any part of this experience? Can you describe a time in your life that music was healing?

3. In the book, the author describes how rhythm is medicine for the body, melody is medicine for the heart, harmony is medicine for the soul, and silence is medicine for the mind. How does each element of music's medicine affect your health?

   What music moves your body?

   What music heals your heart? What is one of your power songs?

   What music touches your soul?

   What music quiets your mind?

4. In chapter 7, the author describes how there is music within us all, claiming that we are a human instrument—*musica humana*. How do you express your inner music?

   If you were an instrument, what would you be?

   What sound or instrument is most like you?

   What sound do you hear when you tune within?

   What does it feel like to sing freely in the shower or play the drum your own way?

   What part of your spirit speaks through music? How is your spirit touched by music?

5. In chapter 8, the author describes the ways in which music can create change on the planet. How do you think music can be used as a tool for healing in the world today?

6. What is one guided practice for both conscious listening and expressing music's medicine that you found most helpful?

Group Experience in Listening and Expressing Music Medicine

Choose one guided practice for conscious listening. Have the group listen to a selection of the playlist together and experience the healing.

Choose one guided practice for expressing music. Invite the group to join together in a healing music experience.

Music Medicine for Music Teachers and Educators

It is more important than ever to bring students into the joy and feeling of musical empowerment. You can create a positive musical experience for your students, whether you teach math, history, or music. Here are some ways that music's medicine can be incorporated into education:

1. *Curriculum development.* You can use a curriculum of experiential education in the classroom. Structure a four-week series using the four elements of music. Select a guided practice for both conscious listening and expressing for each element.

2. *Experiential learning.* The guided practices are tools for experiential learning—both listening and expressing music. Guided practices can be adjusted to group activities. Pair up students or work in small groups of three to four students.

3. *Music in the classroom.* Use music for special school events, such as for Black History Month or other cross-cultural events. Use the orchestrating change playlist (page 173) to highlight world music specific to school themes. Use the rhythm playlist (page 50) when teaching social studies or geography to inspire students to listen to rhythms from around the world. Use the silence playlist (page 128) when teaching earth science to demonstrate music of the tropical rainforest or the practice of singing to the ocean.

4. *Music for learning.* Use music mnemonics in the classroom. After years of watching my sister, Joy Cook, use music in her fourth-grade classes, I've seen how educators can use music recordings to quiet a classroom for homework, study, or reading time, or to energize a classroom after lunch with a rhythm break.

Use the playlists to support your students' learning experiences. The rhythm playlist (page 50) can be a tool to energize students, while the silence playlist (page 128) can provide a peaceful soundscape for schoolwork or reading time. Use the rhythm playlist to provide a beat when learning rules of grammar, math, or spelling. Speak the rules to the beat and watch students retain, repeat, remember, and have fun.

Music Medicine for Counselors and Healing Arts Practitioners

Bringing music into counseling and therapy plays a key role in supporting expression for less verbal clients. From playing music in a waiting area at a counseling office to engaging clients in the guided practices, these tips and tools allow you to incorporate music into your work.

1. *Music listening.* For reiki workers, massage therapists, and energy healers, consider using the silence playlist (page 128) during treatments. The spacious quality of music without a driving beat helps clients relax and release negative thoughts. At the close of a session, consider using a rhythm track (page 50) to help clients be more grounded in their bodies. In addition, be more conscious about the music you play during your healing sessions.

2. *Individual sessions.* For one-on-one counseling, there are many applications of music medicine. As a guided assessment, you can lead a client through the four elements, listening to the music while discussing the aspects that are pertinent to the client's goals. Many guided practices can be used as homework assignments or as a tool to start and end a therapy session. For example, at the start of a session, invite a client to play a drumbeat. Conclude the session with the same exercise and listen for the changes. You may also invite a client to bring a recording of a song that expresses his or her current challenges. For agitated clients, consider playing the soothing music from the silence playlist (page 128) as background sound. Explore how many practices in this book can be useful in counseling.

3. *Couples, support groups, and families.* Sharing music is a powerful healing experience. To bring harmony into groups, you can incorporate ensemble medicine practices, including "Build a Bridge" (page 103), "Create a Herd of Harmony" (page 104), or "Soul Music Sharing" (page 102).

Music Medicine for Coaches and Teambuilding Facilitators

In a sense, coaching can be thought of as helping people change their tune, and teambuilding can be thought of as ensemble medicine. Music is an innovative tool to move people and teams into cathartic experiences through the inherent emotional and healing quality of music.

1. *Life coaching*. The following guided practices are particularly useful when coaching individuals. Because a life coach helps clients find their voices, the melody exercises are particularly resonant with this type of work.

"Finding Your Power Song," chapter 4 (page 74)

"Listening to Your Heart Song," chapter 4 (page 75)

As a client grows, silence practices will help mature and nurture the wisdom within.

"Listening to the Space between the Notes," chapter 6 (page 123)

"Silent Song," chapter 6 (page 125)

2. *Teambuilding*. From learning a rhythm together to igniting the heartbeat of the team, a facilitator helps teams come together in harmony, making the ensemble practices particularly useful.

"Ensemble Ears," chapter 5 (page 102)

"Build a Bridge," chapter 5 (page 103)

"Play Your Part," chapter 5 (page 104)

Start a Music Circle: Orchestrate Change in Your Community

Training Programs for Facilitators

HealthRHYTHMS: remo.com/health

UpBeat Drum Circles: ubdrumcircles.com

Village Music Circles: drumcircle.com

Neurologic Music Therapy Training Institute: colostate.edu/dept/cbrm/institute.htm

Beat the Odds: UCUartsandhealing.net

The Naked Voice: thenakedvoice.com

Vox Mundi Project: voxmundiproject.com

California Institute of Integral Studies—Certificate in Sound, Voice, and Music Healing: ciis.edu/about_ciis/public_programs/certificate_programs/sound_certificate.html

Voices of Eden: voicesofeden.com

Music for People: musicforpeople.org

Recommended Materials

Learning Tools

Christine Stevens, *The Healing Drum Kit* (Boulder, CO: Sounds True).

Wyoma, *African Healing Dance* (Boulder, CO: Sounds True), DVD.

Chantal Pierrat, *Soul Sweat* (Boulder, CO: Sounds True), DVD.

Gabrielle Roth, *Ecstatic Dance: The Gabrielle Roth Video Collection* (Boulder, CO: Sounds True).

Chloë Goodchild, *Your Naked Voice: Sounding from the Source* (Boulder, CO: Sounds True), audio.

Chloë Goodchild, *Awakening through Sound* (Boulder, CO: Sounds True), audio.

Arthur Samuel Joseph, *Sing Your Heart Out* (Boulder, CO: Sounds True), audio.

Silvia Nakkach, *Free Your Voice* (Boulder, CO: Sounds True), book.

Recommended Instruments

Rhythm: Drums and Percussion

Healing drum three-pack: ubdrumcircles.com/products_drumtrio.html

Remo Buffalo drum (12-inch, recommended): remo.com/portal/products/6/120/ww_buffalo_drum.html

Remo Aroma Drum: remo.com/portal/products/684/788/831/ad_aromadrum.html

Remo Ocean Drum: remo.com/portal/products/6/100/ss_ocean_drum.html

Remo Not So Loud Tubano: remo.com/portal/products/6/813/wp_nsl.html

Remo Festival Djembe (medium): remo.com/portal/products/6/28/174/dj_festival.html

Melody

Native American flutes: highspirits.com

Harmony

Strumstick (three-string guitar with no wrong notes; key of D is recommended): feeltone.usa.com/feeltone/the_sansula_renaissance.html

"Christine Stevens and Inspirational Strumstick": strumstick.com/html_pages/Christine%20Stevens.htm

Silence: Tibetan Singing Bowls and Bells

Tibetan Singing Bowls: sacredsoundgongbath.com/Sacred_Sound_Gong_Bath/Singing_Bowls.html

How to play a singing bowl: youtube.com/watch?v=LvsWWVVi-Nc

Movies

Discover the Gift

El Sistema

Favela Rising

The Singing Revolution

The Visitor

The Music Instinct: Science and Song

As It Is in Heaven

The Piano

I Know I'm Not Alone

Singing in Baghdad: A Musical Mission of Peace

Afghan Star

About the Author

Christine Stevens, MSW, MT-BC, is a music therapist and author of *The Healing Drum Kit* and *The Art and Heart of Drum Circles*. The founder of UpBeat Drum Circles and wellness consultant to Remo Drum Company's HealthRHYTHMS, she has worked with many Fortune 500 companies, Katrina survivors, students at Grond Zero, and led the first drum-circle training in Iraq. Christine lives in Encinitas, California. For more information on Christine and her work, see ubdrumcircles.com. Visit ubdrumcircles.com/music medicine. Contact Christine at info@ubdrumcircles.com.

About Sounds True

Sounds True is a multimedia publisher whose mission is to inspire and support personal transformation and spiritual awakening. Founded in 1985 and located in Boulder, Colorado, we work with many of the leading spiritual teachers, thinkers, healers, and visionary artists of our time. We strive with every title to preserve the essential "living wisdom" of the author or artist. It is our goal to create products that not only provide information to a reader or listener, but that also embody the quality of a wisdom transmission.

For those seeking genuine transformation, Sounds True is your trusted partner. At SoundsTrue.com you will find a wealth of free resources to support your journey, including exclusive weekly audio interviews, free downloads, interactive learning tools, and other special savings on all our titles.

To listen to a podcast interview with Sounds True publisher Tami Simon and author Christine Stevens, please visit SoundsTrue.com/MusicMedicinePodcast.

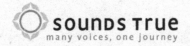

Printed in the USA
CPSIA information can be obtained
at www.ICGtesting.com
LVHW030212130624
783117LV00016B/538